TRANSGENDER HEALTH ISSUES

Sarah Boslaugh

Health and Medical Issues Today

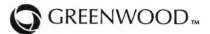
GREENWOOD™

An Imprint of ABC-CLIO, LLC
Santa Barbara, California • Denver, Colorado

Library of Congress Cataloging-in-Publication Data

Names: Boslaugh, Sarah, author.
Title: Transgender health issues / Sarah Boslaugh.
Description: Santa Barbara, California : Greenwood/ABC-CLIO, LLC, [2018] |
    Series: Health and medical issues today | Includes bibliographical
    references and index.
Identifiers: LCCN 2018014992 (print) | LCCN 2018017746 (ebook) |
    ISBN 9781440858888 (ebook) | ISBN 9781440858871 (print : alk. paper)
Subjects: LCSH: Transgender people—Health and hygiene. | Transgender
    people—Social aspects.
Classification: LCC RA564.87 (ebook) | LCC RA564.87 .B67 2018 (print) |
    DDC 362.1086/7—dc23
LC record available at https://lccn.loc.gov/2018014992

ISBN: 978-1-4408-5887-1 (print)
      978-1-4408-5888-8 (ebook)

22 21 20 19 18   1 2 3 4 5

This book is also available as an eBook.

Greenwood
An Imprint of ABC-CLIO, LLC

ABC-CLIO, LLC
130 Cremona Drive, P.O. Box 1911
Santa Barbara, California 93116-1911
www.abc-clio.com

This book is printed on acid-free paper ∞

Manufactured in the United States of America

CONTENTS

SERIES FOREWORD

Every day, the public is bombarded with information on developments in medicine and health care. Whether it is on the latest techniques in treatment or research, or on concerns over public health threats, this information directly affects the lives of people more than almost any other issue. Although there are many sources for understanding these topics—from websites and blogs to newspapers and magazines—students and ordinary citizens often need one resource that makes sense of the complex health and medical issues affecting their daily lives.

The *Health and Medical Issues Today* series provides just such a one-stop resource for obtaining a solid overview of the most controversial areas of health care in the 21st century. Each volume addresses one topic and provides a balanced summary of what is known. These volumes provide an excellent first step for students and lay people interested in understanding how health care works in our society today.

Each volume is broken into several parts to provide readers and researchers with easy access to the information they need:

- Part I provides overview chapters on background information—including chapters on such areas as the historical, scientific, medical, social, and legal issues involved—that a citizen needs to intelligently understand the topic.
- Part II provides capsule examinations of the most heated contemporary issues and debates and analyzes in a balanced manner the viewpoints held by various advocates in the debates.
- Part III provides case studies that show examples of the concepts discussed in the previous sections.

A selection of reference material, such as a timeline of important events and a directory of organizations, serves as the best next step in learning about the topic at hand.

The *Health and Medical Issues Today* series strives to provide readers with all the information needed to begin making sense of some of the most important debates going on in the world today. The series includes volumes on such topics as stem-cell research, obesity, gene therapy, alternative medicine, organ transplantation, mental health, and more.

INTRODUCTION

To be transgender is to have a gender identity that does not correspond to the identity assigned you at birth. This is an unusual state of being in a world in which the vast majority of people never give gender identity a second thought—they are identified at birth as male or female, grow up to be boys or girls, then become men or women, all in concordance with their original gender identification. When you've always taken something as basic as gender identity for granted, it can come as a shock to learn that it's not that simple for everyone.

People generally resist having their basic assumptions about the world challenged, and the very existence of transgender people constitutes a challenge to a whole host of often unstated assumptions about gender, beginning with the belief that there are exactly two genders and everyone fitting neatly into one or the other. Not everyone appreciates having so simple and tidy a worldview overturned, and while some respond with curiosity and a desire for more knowledge, others react with defensiveness, fear, and hatred. One goal of this book is to provide everyone, no matter their current understanding of transgender issues, with information that will help them move toward a better understanding and acceptance of transgender people, as well as an appreciation of how complex issues of gender identity can be. Another goal is to provide information and resources to people of all ages who are actively seeking information about transgender issues, whether to help clarify their own situation, to help a friend, or simply to become a better informed citizen of the world.

This is a book about transgender health issues, so it includes information about specific health concerns of transgender people, such as the many options for the gender transition (gender affirmation) process and the health risks associated with certain procedures. However, health is not simply about what happens in the doctor's office, the medical clinic, or the hospital. In this volume, health is broadly defined by drawing on the famous formulation from the preamble to the constitution of the World Health Organization: "Health is a state of complete physical, mental and social well-being and not merely the absence of disease or infirmity."

Transgender people are a small minority of the world's population and are often victims of discrimination and persecution. Any consideration of transgender health must therefore take into account the stress and strain that comes from living in the world of as part of a misunderstood and sometimes despised minority group. It must also consider the impact of widespread discrimination against transgender people, and the very real risk of being assaulted or even killed due to one's transgender status.

It would be a mistake to dwell only on the negative, however. In recent years we've seen a host of transgender people, both celebrities and private citizens, come forward to identify themselves and tell their stories to the public. Young people today seem more willing to accept gender identity as a continuum rather than a simple binary, are less concerned with policing other people's choices regarding gender expression, and are simply more willing to embrace the variety of human existence rather than forcing people into a preexisting schema. Many governments and private entities are also beginning to acknowledge the diversity of gender identities that exist in the world, and enacting laws and policies to protect the rights of those who may not fit the gender binary model. Education is a key factor in overcoming prejudice, and *Transgender Health Issues* hopes to make a contribution to that effort while at the same time empowering transgender people and their allies with knowledge that will help them live their best lives.

PART I

Overview

CHAPTER 1

What Does It Mean to Be Transgender?

One of the most obvious characteristics of human beings is how variable we are—while we certainly have much in common, we also differ from each other in many ways. We are all human, but we are also all unique. While this has always been the case, it was not until the late 20th century that it became common to acknowledge the fact that one of the ways that people vary is in their gender identity. While for centuries the simple male/female dichotomy was assumed to be adequate, and it was assumed that gender was determined by physical characteristics present at birth, we now know that human gender identity is far more complex than previously understood, and that an individual's gender identity can change over time over the course of their life. This chapter will set the stage for chapters to follow by discussing some key terms used through the book, reviewing what is known about the number and characteristics of the transgender population in the United States and worldwide, and introducing the topic of intersectionality, which is key to understanding the lives of many transgender people.

SOME BASIC DEFINITIONS

The study of minority sexualities and divergent sexual identities is relatively recent, and the terminology used within this field is still evolving. Certain terms that used to be commonly used are now considered offensive, while new terms are regularly introduced that may be unfamiliar even to people who work in this field. Every effort has been made in this book to use terms that are accurate but not offensive, but because people differ as to the appropriateness of some terminology, it's possible that some of the terminology may seem inappropriate or even disparaging to some individuals. Be assured that there is no intention to give offense.

Human sexuality and gender identity are complex topics, so it's not surprising that the same term might be defined differently in different studies or by different people: for instance, classifying a person as heterosexual might be based on their sexual behavior, their sexual desires, their self-perceived gender or sexual identity, how others perceive their gender or sexual identity, or some combination of these or other factors. Confusion may arise when different writers or researchers use the same word with different meanings. In the interests of clarity, this section will define and discuss some basic terminology that will be used in this book, based on the terminology used in the 2011 report "The Health of Lesbian, Gay, Bisexual, and Transgender People: Building a Foundation for Better Understanding" released by the Institute of Medicine.

Scientists distinguish between *sex*, which is a biological construct, and *gender*, which is a cultural construct. Sex includes physiological characteristics such as genetic makeup, hormones, and anatomical and physiological characteristics (e.g., genitalia, skeleton, facial and body hair), and an infant's sex is typically assigned at birth on the basis of external genitalia. Gender includes aspects such as experience, personality, and patterns of behavior, and the meanings they carry in a particular society or culture. While sexual characteristics are more likely to be commonly defined as either male or female across many societies, the gendered meaning of behaviors, personality, and other types of expression often differs from one society to another. An individual's gender identity may be consonant with their gender identity as assigned at birth, or it may differ from that assigned identity.

Gender identity refers to an individual's sense of being male, female, or another gender; the latter can include categories such as *genderqueer* or *gender nonconforming*, both of which may signify that the individual rejects the binary male/female classification of gender. The adjectives *masculine* and *feminine* in this context refer to qualities, behaviors, appearances, and so on, that are considered appropriate to men or women in a specific cultural context. For instance, in a given society or culture, speaking in an aggressive manner might be considered a masculine trait, and deferring to others might be considered a feminine trait, while in a different society or culture the opposite might be true. *Gender expression* refers to behaviors, clothing, personality characteristics, and other aspects of an individual that are defined in their culture as either masculine or feminine. *Gender role conformity* means adhering to the gender expressions deemed culturally appropriate for one's sex. As with the terms *masculine* and *feminine*, exactly what constitutes gender role conformity is not universal but rather is defined with reference to a particular society or culture.

Gender dysphoria refers to an individual's sense of discomfort with the sex assigned to them at birth. This discomfort can take many forms, from the individual's unease with their current primary or secondary sexual characteristics to a more general sense that the gender assigned at birth is not appropriate. Gender dysphoria is described in the *Diagnostic and Statistical Manual of Mental Disorders* (*DSM-5*) of the American Psychiatric Association, which specifies criteria for diagnosing this condition in children, adolescents, and adults. *Gender identity disorder* was a term used in the previous *Diagnostic and Statistical Manual of Mental Disorders* (*DSM-IV*) for a similar condition, and the term *gender identity disorder* is also used in the tenth edition of the *International Statistical Classification of Diseases and Related Problems* (*ICD-10*), a medical classification list produced by the World Health Organization.

Transgender is a broad term used to describe a number of individuals who feel that their gender assigned at birth is not correct. This term is contrasted with the term *cisgender* (sometimes abbreviated to "cis"), which refers to individuals whose gender identity matches the gender they were assigned to at birth. Behaviors can also be described as transgender: for instance, some people consider cross-dressing (wearing clothing, hairstyles, makeup, etc., associated in one's culture with the opposite sex) as a transgender behavior. However, the cross-dressing doesn't make a person transgender because the behavior itself tells you nothing about the motivation behind it or the meaning the behavior holds for the individual. For instance, transvestites dress at least some of the time as a member of the opposite sex, and drag queens and kings appear as members of the opposite sex in public performances, but it is not necessary for members of either group to experience any incongruity between their birth sex and their gender identity. For the sake of clarity, within this book the term *transgender* will be reserved for those who feel that the gender they were assigned at birth does not coincide with their felt gender identity, without regard to whether they have taken any actions toward bringing their bodies into congruence with their gender identity. In other words, if someone says they are transgender, they are, and questions such as whether they have or intend to undergo surgery or hormone treatment are irrelevant.

Transsexual is a similar term used in some contexts to refer to people whose gender identity does not correspond with their sex as assigned at birth. As with the term *transgender*, classifying someone as transsexual is based on their internal gender identity being out of congruence with the sex they were assigned at birth, and does not require that the individual have taken any steps toward bringing them into congruence. Two other terms often used when describing transgender or transsexual people are *male-to-female* or *transwoman*, which refers to a person identified as male at birth, but whose gender identity is female, and *female-to-male* or *transman*, which refers to someone identified as female at birth but whose gender identity is male.

How Are Sex and Gender Defined?

There are a number of ways to define an individual's sex and gender. For most people, all the common systems (chromosomes, physical appearance, and self-identification) produce the same result, the person is clearly either male or female, and their gender identification matches their biological sex. For some people, however, one or more of these systems of identifying gender is not consonant with the others. In some cases, the discrepancy is minor, and the person is happy with the gender they were assigned at birth. In other cases, the person may decide that their birth gender is incorrect, and they are actually of the other gender, or that some other term, such as *gender neutral, gender nonconforming*, or *genderqueer*, better describes them.

Chromosomes

One method of determining who is male and who is female is by their chromosomal makeup. Most humans have 23 pairs of chromosomes (46 in total), including 22 pairs of autosomes (body chromosomes, as distinguished from sex chromosomes) and 1 pair of allosomes (sex chromosomes). Sex chromosomes are classified as X or Y, and the XY sex-determination system is used to describe the sex of individuals at the chromosomal level, so that individuals with two X chromosomes are classified as female and those with one X and one Y are designated as male. The chromosomal makeup of most males is therefore described as 46,XY (46 chromosomes, including one X and one Y sex chromosomes), and most females as 46,XX (46 chromosomes, including two X sex chromosomes).

While the chromosomal makeup of most people fits one category or the other, several variants exist in the population. Some people have some cells that are XX and some that are XY, a condition known as mosaicism, and others (generally estimated as a few per 1,000 births) may have different chromosomal makeups. For instance, some individuals have a single sex chromosome (45,X or 45,Y, also referred to as 45,X0 and 45,Y0), some have three sex chromosomes (47,XXX, 47,XXY, etc.), and some males are born 46,XX and some females 46,XY. In most cases, the chromosomal makeup of an individual matches with their external appearance and sense of gender identity, but this is not true for everyone.

One reason people outside the medical community may be aware of the existence of chromosomal variants is the publicity afforded to the cases of some female athletes who were disqualified from competition due to their nonstandard chromosomal makeup. Typically, these athletes had lived their entire lives as females and had never had any reason to suspect that there was anything unusual about their bodies and yet were not allowed to compete as women due to a lab test indicating their chromosomal makeup was something other than 46,XX. Because we now recognize that gender has social and psychological aspects, and that there is more variety in chromosomal makeup than was previously believed, the simple statement that females are XX and males are XY is no longer accepted in the scientific community.

Some variations in chromosomal makeup are common enough to have been studied in detail. Persons with Turner syndrome (45,X) are phenotypically female, meaning that their observable sex-based characteristics are those associated with females, although they are sterile, tend to be short, and lack prominent female secondary sexual characteristics. Persons with three X chromosomes (47,XXX) are taller and more slender than average, have normal development of female sexual traits, and are fertile. Individuals with Klinefelter syndrome (47,XXY) are phenotypically male but infertile, produce small amounts of testosterone, and have incompletely developed male secondary sex characteristics. Males with the XXY makeup have higher than usual amounts of testosterone, are taller than average, and are usually fertile.

Even if an individual's chromosomes are 46,XX or 46,XY, a medical condition may affect the way inherited sex characteristics are expressed. For instance, individuals born 46,XX (typically female chromosomes) with congenital adrenal hyperplasia (CAH) will have a deficiency of cortisol, which may result in incomplete female sex differentiation and an outwardly male appearance. Individuals born with typically male chromosomes (46,XY) but who have androgen insensitivity syndrome (AIS) will develop external female genitalia and breasts because their body does not respond to androgens (male hormones) but does respond to estrogen (a female hormone). Such individuals are likely to have been raised as females and to have a female gender identity, despite having the chromosomal makeup typical of a man.

Physical Appearance

Gender is typically assigned at birth, based on the appearance of the baby's genitals: "It's a boy!" or "It's a girl!" is typically proclaimed without any knowledge of the baby's chromosomal makeup. For most infants, the genitals and chromosomal makeup coincide, but in some cases it does not. For instance, as mentioned earlier, a baby with AIS has the outward genitalia of a female but the chromosomal makeup of a male. AIS may not be diagnosed until puberty, when the individual does not begin to have menstrual periods as expected.

Similarly, a baby with CAH has the chromosomal makeup (46,XX) typical of a female but may be born with ambiguous genitalia due to being exposed to high levels of androgens before birth. However, most CAH females have typical internal female reproductive organs (ovaries, fallopian tubes, and uterus), and most identify as female, so their sexual identification matches their chromosomal makeup. A small proportion of persons with CAH have the typical male chromosomal makeup (46,XY). Some may be born with ambiguous genitalia, but for most there are no indications of CAH until they begin to experience premature onset of puberty (e.g., early appearance of pubic hair and deepened voice).

Psychosocial Identity

Gender identity refers to how a person perceives and experiences themselves—as male, female, or some other category—and does not bear a necessary relation to either chromosomal makeup or genitalia. The psychosocial aspects of gender identity and expression are newer topics for study than are the medical aspects of gender (chromosomes and genitalia), but the importance of this part of gender identity is increasingly accepted by the medical and psychological communities. Because gender identity is internal, an individual is the sole expert on their own gender identity, and it may or may not conform to the gender category they have been assigned. In addition, gender identity can change over a person's life course and is independent of other issues such as sexual identity or sexual behavior, so a transgender person could be straight, gay, bisexual, asexual, or prefer some other term to describe their sexuality.

HOW MANY TRANSGENDER PEOPLE ARE THERE?

It's currently impossible to answer the question of how many transgender people there are in the world because no survey or census has been conducted that could answer that question. Most survey-based studies of transgender people have been conducted on small, nonprobability samples that make it impossible to generalize from the study sample to the larger population (in order words, one cannot use the information from the sample to make statistical statements about the total transgender population). The few probability samples that have collected information about transgender people tend to be limited, requiring researchers to extrapolate from the available data to estimate the number of transgender people within a given population or geographic area, and such estimation requires making assumptions than can lead to inaccurate results. In the future, better samples may be drawn and more accurate surveys conducted, and in the mean time we will interpret any generalizations based on surveys with a knowledge of their limitations.

Intersex Conditions

Intersex is a culturally constructed category created to accommodate a system of classifying individuals into exactly two categories, male or female, a system sometimes referred to as the gender binary. Nature, in contrast, produces organisms (including people) with a variety of sexual, chromosomal, and other characteristics. For this reason, some researchers prefer to think of gender as a continuum rather than a set of distinct categories. In this point of view, there is no absolute definition of "male" and "female" in nature, so any such definitions are created by people and are therefore culturally specific rather than absolute.

While some prefer the term *disorders of sex development* or DSD, the term *intersex* is still used in medical discourse and by organizations such as the World Health Organization. Someone born with an intersex condition may have any sexual preference and any gender identity, so that an intersex person is not necessarily transgender.

Examples of conditions that might cause a baby to be classified as intersex include ambiguous external genitals (i.e., genitals that are not easily classified as either male or female), unusual or incomplete development of internal reproductive organs, abnormalities of the sex chromosomes, inconsistency between external genitals and internal reproductive organs, abnormal production of sex-related hormones, and unusual response or lack of response to sex hormones.

The lack of agreed-upon parameters for what constitutes an anomaly (e.g., at what measurement does a penis become abnormally small, which chromosomal abnormalities should be included within the category of intersex) makes it difficult to determine how common intersex births are. The Intersex Society of North America estimates that about 1 in every

100 births differ in some way from standard definitions of male or female, with about 1 in every 1,500 to 2,000 children born with noticeably atypical genitalia. This category does not include all types of difference (e.g., it does not consider chromosomal abnormalities that do not result in external differences in genitalia), demonstrating another difficulty in determining how many people are born with intersex characteristics—exactly which characteristics are you considering? Including chromosomal and other conditions within the definition of intersex not surprisingly raises the estimated number of such births, with some estimates running as high as 1.7 percent of all births (17 intersex births per 1,000 births), although that estimate includes conditions that many researchers do not consider intersex.

United States

Two estimates based on large-scale surveys are available to estimate the number of transgender people in the United States. In 2011, Gary J. Gates used data from surveys conducted in California and Massachusetts to estimate that 0.3 percent of the U.S. adult population (about 700,000 people) identified as transgender. In 2016, Andrew R. Flores and colleagues used data from the Behavioral Risk Factor Surveillance System (BRFSS), a survey conducted annually by the Centers for Disease Control and Prevention (CDC) and state health departments, to estimate that about 0.6 percent of American adults identify as transgender (about 1.4 million people).

Flores's estimate is based on data from 19 states that used an optional module including the question, "Do you consider yourself to be transgender?" If that question was answered in the affirmative, the interviewer followed-up with the question, "Do you consider yourself to be male-to-female, female-to-male, or gender nonconforming?" Data from these states was then statistically adjusted to estimate the number of transgender people in each state and in the United States as a whole.

By their calculations, the state with the highest percentage of people identifying as transgender is Hawaii (0.78%), followed by California (0.76%) and New Mexico (0.75%). The states estimated to have the lowest percentage of transgender people were Wyoming (0.32%), Iowa (0.31%), and North Dakota (0.30%). They also calculated that persons in the 18–24 years age group were the most likely to identify as transgender (0.66%), followed by people in the 25–64 years age group (0.58%) and that transgender identification was least likely in people 65 and older (0.50%).

Other Countries

There is currently no way to know the exact number of transgender people in the world. However, several recent population-based studies, summarized by Sam Winter and colleagues, have produced estimates in the range of 0.5 percent to 1.2 percent transgender people in the population studied. Three of these studies were conducted in Europe, one in the United States, and one in New Zealand, and all used large samples (from 1,832 to 9,950 subjects). However, particular care should be used in interpreting these results on a global level, since much less is known about the transgender population in larger regions of the world, including Africa, Asia, the Middle East, the Caribbean, and Latin America.

According to a 2014 report by Amnesty International, studies that identify as transgender those individuals who had undergone hormonal or surgical treatments related to their transgender status, or who had sought legal recognition of a gender change, place the estimate at about 30,000 transgender people living in the European Union. However, this estimate excludes the many transgender people who have not sought hormonal or surgical treatments and or legal recognition of a gender change. Other studies that use a more inclusive definition of transgender as those who do not completely identify with the sex they were classified as at birth place the estimate at about 1.5 million transgender individuals.

A population-based study in Massachusetts by Kerith J. Conron and colleagues found that about 0.5 percent (one-half of 1%) of the state's population was transgender. It is not known whether this same percentage can be applied to other populations, because transgender people might move from a region in which they felt discriminated against or unsafe to a different region where they felt their safety and rights were better protected. However, using the 0.5 percent standard, this would equate to, for instance, about 181,432 transgender people in Canada (using StatCan's population estimate of 36,286,400) and 2.54 million transgender people in the European Union (using the European Union's 2016 population estimate of 508 million). Using a world population estimate of 7.4 billion, this would equate to about 37 million transgender people across all countries.

CHARACTERISTICS OF THE TRANSGENDER COMMUNITY

Although there are few surveys providing even an estimate of the total transgender population, there are more that have studied the characteristics of specific populations of transgender people. Most such surveys are neither randomized nor population based, making them descriptive of a particular group of people but not providing sufficient information to allow generalizations about the transgender population as a whole. However, they still provide useful information for understanding the transgender community and for providing services for transgender individuals. Such surveys also increase our understanding of the diversity that exists within the transgender community and help us understand how intersectionality (discussed in the next section) can affect the life of transgender individuals.

United States

The best single source of general information about the adult transgender community in the United States is the 2016 report of the National Center for Transgender Equality, written by Sandy E. James and colleagues, based on a survey conducted with 27,715 transgender adults from all 50 states, the District of Columbia, U.S. overseas military bases, and American Samoa, Guam, and Puerto Rico. This survey was conducted online and includes the self-reported experiences of a broad sample of transgender people. While this study is not based on a random sample, it was weighted by race and ethnicity, and to correct for a disproportion number of people who said their age was 18, in order to make results from the sample correspond more closely to the U.S. population. Additional weights for age and educational attainment were also applied to data sensitive to those variables, including individual and household income.

Sample respondents were more likely to be members of minority groups than is true in the general population: only 62.2 percent were white, with 16.6 percent Hispanic, 12.6 percent black, 5.1 percent Asian, and the rest multiracial, Middle Eastern, or American Indian. The age of respondents in the sample ranged from 18 to 87 years, and respondents were generally younger than the U.S. population, with 42 percent aged 18 to 24, 42 percent aged 25 to 44, 14 percent aged 45 to 64, and 2 percent aged 65 and older. A disproportionate number indicated they were 18 years old, the minimum age to take the survey, so the sample was weighted so that it better reflects the distribution of the U.S. population as a whole.

More than one-third (35%) of the respondents indicated that their gender identity was nonbinary or genderqueer, with 33 percent indicating their identity was that of a transgender woman, 29 percent that of a transgender man, and 3 percent that of a cross-dresser. Most said they began to feel that their gender designation at birth was not correct by age 10 or younger (including 32% who had such feelings at age 5 or younger), while

21 percent reporting first experiencing such feelings between age 11 and 15, 13 percent between age 16 and 20, 4 percent between age 21 and 25, and 2 percent when they were aged 26 or older.

Income data was weighted by age and educational attainment as well as race and ethnicity because age and educational attainment are known to be related to income. Looking at individual income in the sample as compared to national averages, those in the sample were disproportionately lower income, but were slightly less likely to report having no income. The difference was even starker in comparing household incomes, although this statistic was not corrected for size of household. Nearly one-third (29%) of the sample reported living in poverty, more than twice the percentage in the United States as a whole (14%). In contrast, the sample was generally better educated than the U.S. population as a whole, with only 18 percent of those aged 18 to 24 having a high school diploma or less (as compared to 44% of the general population), 65 percent having an associate's degree or having attended college without receiving a bachelor's degree (as compared to 46% in the general population), and 17 percent having a bachelor's degree or higher (as compared to 10% of the general population).

Benjamin Cerf Harris used data from the Social Security Administration to identify those who made changes (in first or middle name, and/or sex code) consistent with gender transition. He found such changes as early as 1936, with changes more common in later years, particularly since 1970: of the 135,367 who changed their information in ways consistent with gender transition, 89,667 were still alive during the 2010 U.S. Census. While this is likely a vast undercount of the number of transgender people in the United States (it would equate to a transgender rate of about 300ths of 1%), linking this data to data from the 2010 Census allowed Harris to provide useful information describing individuals who met Harris's criteria.

Most people changed both pieces of information (name[s] and sex code) concurrently, but 27 percent changed their name first and their sex code later. Those who transitioned from female to male were more likely to change their name first, then their sex code later (31%), as compared to those who transitioned from male to female (24%). Most began making changes consistent with gender transition in their mid-30s, although transgender women tend to begin making these changes at a somewhat older age. The percentage of such individuals who were black or Hispanic was also higher than has been found in some other studies, and individuals making these changes were not evenly distributed across the United States. Instead, it was most common for people living in the states of Oregon,

Washington, and Vermont (all with rates from 7.7 to 10.6 per 100,000 population) to make changes, and they were less common in a number of southern and western states that had rates between 1.4 per 100,000 and 3.3 per 100,000.

Canada

In 2011, Trans PULSE undertook a survey with 433 individuals aged 16 or older who live, work, or receive health care in Ontario. As reported by Todd Coleman and colleagues, 54 percent of those identifying as transgender said their transition was from female to male, and 47 percent male to female (adding up to 101% due to rounding). Only 6 percent reported having a medically recognized intersex diagnosis. Twenty percent reported that their gender identity was both male and female, neither male nor female, or fluid; apart from those individuals, most had a gender identity consonant with their chosen gender status (no male-to-female individuals identified their gender identity as masculine, and only 2% of female-to-male individuals identified their gender identity as feminine).

Overall, 59 percent said they first realized that their gender identity did not match their body before the age of 10, while 21 percent first had that recognition between 10 and 14 years, 13 percent between 15 and 19 years, 7 percent between 20 and 29 years, and only 1 percent at age 30 or later. Similar patterns were observed for female-to-male and male-to-female individuals, with the latter somewhat more likely to notice the discrepancy between body and gender at a younger age. Just under half (48%) were currently living full time in their felt gender, with 30 percent living in that gender part-time, and 22 percent not at all. One-fourth reported they had completed a medical transition, 24 percent were in process of transition, 28 percent were planning their transition, and the remainder were unsure, not planning to transition, or felt the concept of transition did not apply to them.

The 2015 report "Being Safe, Being Me," based on the Canadian Trans Youth Health Survey, provides substantial information about the young transgender Canadians (aged 14–25) who took part in the survey. The survey used a voluntary sample and was not weighted, so should not be considered representative of the Canadian transgender youth population but does provide an interesting description of those who participated in the survey. Most of the participants (74%) identified as white, with 10 percent aboriginal, 5 percent East Asian, and the remainder other ethnic or cultural backgrounds. Most (87%) had lived in Canada their entire lives, while only 2 percent reported immigrating to Canada within the past two years.

Most (83%) reported living in their felt gender at least some of the time, with 45 percent living in their felt gender full time. Older respondents were more likely than younger to be living in their felt gender full time, and those living in British Columbia were the most likely (53%) to be living in their felt gender full time, while those in Ontario were least likely (29%) to be living full time in their felt gender.

Respondents were allowed to choose multiple categories for their gender identity. The categories most often selected were queer (49%) or pan sexual (35%), followed by "I am transgender and identify in some other way" (17%), bisexual (17%), straight or heterosexual (14%), gay (13%), lesbian (12%), not sure or questioning (11%), asexual (10%), and Two Spirit (4%). Among aboriginal trans youth, 28 percent identified as Two Spirit.

Europe

Results from the largest sample of transgender individuals in Europe are contained in the "European Union Lesbian, Gay, Bisexual and Transgender Survey." The basis of this report is data collected through a non-random online survey conducted with 93,079 individuals residing in one of the European Union countries and weighted so the sample population from each country is proportionate to each country's population, and the distribution and the relative size of each group (lesbian, gay, bisexual, and transgender) within a country is proportionate to the country's population. The latter weighting was performed to correct for the fact that previous studies have found that gay men are disproportionately likely to respond to surveys; since the number or percentage of individuals in each group is not known, as a compromise it was assumed to be the same in each country.

Seven percent of this sample self-identified as transgender; after weighting, transgender people constituted 8 percent of the sample. Among the transgender respondents, about two-thirds (66%) were designated male at birth. Most of the transgender sample described themselves as bisexual (27%) or gay (28%), with about 14 percent describing themselves as heterosexual or not agreeing with any of the categories offered (which included transgender, transsexual, woman with a transsexual past, man with a transsexual past, gender variant, cross-dresser, or queer). Sexual attraction varied within the transgender group, with 36 percent reporting that they were sexually attracted by men, 31 percent by women, and 29 percent by both men and women.

The sample was not weighted to make it correspond more nearly to the age distributions of the countries surveyed, so particular caution should be exercised when generalizing about factors such as education and income (both usually related to age) to any larger population. Of the transgender individuals who responded to the survey, 30 percent were aged 18–24, 39 percent were aged 25–39, 24 percent were aged 40–54, and 8 percent were aged 55 or older. Three percent of transgender respondents had only a primary education, 30 percent had completed secondary education (high school or the equivalent), 16 percent had postsecondary education other than college or university, 48 percent had higher education in a college or university, and 3 percent reported some other level of education. Fifty percent said they were employed in paid work, 24 percent were students, 13 percent were unemployed, 4 percent were retired, 3 percent were in voluntary or unpaid work, and 6 percent were otherwise not working (e.g., disabled, on long-term sick leave). Over one-third (36%) had household incomes in the lowest quartile (i.e., the lowest 25 percent) for their country, 25 percent were in the second quartile, 20 percent were in the third quartile, and 19 percent were in the upper quartile.

Over half (59%) of transgender respondents reported living in a city, 21 percent in a town, 10 percent in the suburbs, 9 percent in a country village, and 2 percent in the countryside. Thirty percent lived alone, 30 percent in a household with 2 people, 18 percent in a household with three people, 14 percent in a household with 4 people, and 9 percent in a household with five or more people (the question was not applicable for 1% of the respondents). Forty-eight percent said they were not currently in a relationship, 24 percent said they were in a relationship but did not live with their partner or spouse, and 29 percent lived with their partner or spouse. Fifteen percent said they were married or in a registered partnership (i.e., the partnership was recognized by their country), 74 percent were single, 7 percent divorced, 2 percent separated, and 1 percent widowed. Sixteen percent said they lived in a household including at least one child.

INTERSECTIONALITY

The term *intersectionality* was coined by Kimberlé Crenshaw to refer to the ways power structures interact to affect the lives of black women, and the need to understand how multiple types of discrimination can affect a person's life. For instance, a black woman could be subject to discrimination based on her race, based on her gender, or both types of discrimination could interact. This type of thinking contrasts with the traditional legal approach, which looks at each type of discrimination separately. In addition, intersectionality explicitly includes the notion that a person's life experience may be affected by their multiple social identities (so a single individual could have social identities based on gender, race, sexual preference, social class, immigration status, and so on), so that the experience within any group defined by a single characteristic (e.g., all women) will actually include a diversity of experiences that are affected by other characteristics of the individuals in question. For instance, black women and white women may have common experiences based on their gender, but also divergent experiences based on other characteristics, such as race.

Intersectionality is an important concept to use when thinking about transgender people, because of the diversity among transgender people and the fact that other social identities may interact with an individual's transgender status to affect their life in various ways. This is a difficult topic to research because the number of transgender individuals in almost any population is small relative to the size of the population as a whole, making breakdowns by different categories difficult. In addition, questions about transgender status are not included in most major population-based surveys, so that the information we have about intersectionalities in the transgender communities typically comes from smaller, nonrandom studies focused on particular subpopulations, making it impossible to generalize to the entire population. However, even small, nonrandom studies can provide useful information about the experiences of transgender people.

A 2011 report by Jaime M. Grant, Lisa A. Mottet, and Justin Tanis, "Injustice at Every Turn: A Report of the National Transgender Discrimination Survey," provides substantial information about the discrimination faced by transgender people in the United States, and of how that discrimination can interact with an individual's other social identities to increase the discrimination they suffer. This report, conducted under the auspices of the National Center for Transgender Equality and the National Gay and Lesbian Task Force, gathered information from over 6,400 transgender and gender nonconforming individuals from all 50 U.S. states plus the District of Columbia, Puerto Rico, Guam, and the U.S. Virgin Islands, making the sample studied one of the largest and most diverse in the field of transgender research.

Grant and colleagues found that discrimination and low quality of life were common experiences of transgender people, that matters were even worse for transgender people of color as compared to transgender white people, and that black transgender individuals came out the worst of any group studied. This is a textbook case of intersectionality: transgender people are discriminated against in the United States, as are black people, so someone who is both black and transgender is likely to suffer even more discrimination than a person with only one of those characteristics. Examples of the lower quality of life experienced by transgender people, as compared to the general U.S. population, include a much higher risk of living in extreme poverty, much higher risk of attempting suicide, high rates experiencing of harassment and assault, and twice the rate of unemployment of cisgender people.

Although discrimination and disadvantage were common experiences for transgender people, other social factors often combined to make it even more common for specific subgroups. For instance, the unemployment rate for the general U.S. population was 7 percent, as compared to 14 percent in the transgender sample, However, there was significant variability in unemployment by race and ethnicity within the transgender sample: black transgender people had the highest rate of unemployment, 28 percent, followed by 24 percent of transgender American Indians and 18 percent of Hispanic or multiracial transgender people. In contrast, the unemployment rate for Asian transgender people was 10 percent, and for white transgender people 12 percent, both above the average for the population, but much lower than for other racial and ethnic groups in the sample. Similarly, while 22 percent of the transgender sample reported being harassed by the police, the rate was much highest for black (38%) and multiracial (36%) individuals, as compared to 29 percent for Asian individuals, 24 percent for American Indian individuals, 23 percent for Hispanic individuals, and 18 percent for white individuals.

A follow-up study by James and colleagues, conducted in 2015, found similar patterns of discrimination. For instance, the unemployment rate in the transgender sample was 15 percent, three times higher than in the U.S. population as a whole (5%). However, unemployment was much higher among transgender people of color, with the highest rates reported by people from the Middle East (35%), followed by America Indians (23%), multiracial individuals (22%), Hispanics (21%), and blacks (20%). In contrast, the lowest rates of unemployment within the transgender sample were found among white people (12%) and Asians (10%).

Other studies have also found that intersectionality plays a significant role in the experiences of transgender people. For instance, Rodrigo

Aguayo-Romero, Natalie M. Alizaga, and Courtney Glickman report that studies have found the rate of intimate partner violence (IPV) as high as 25 percent among transgender people, with rates even higher among transgender people of color. Transgender people of color also report experiencing more discrimination in other aspects of their life, including discrimination within healthcare settings, suggesting that the rate of IPV may be even higher. Transgender people who are undocumented (i.e., were born in another country and do not have the legal right to be in the United States) also suffer high rates of IPV than do those legally allowed to stay in the United States.

CHAPTER 2

A Brief History of Transgender People

Although the term *transgender* is of relatively recent origin, people whose sense of gender did not conform to the societal standards of their day have probably existed throughout human history. Although the historical record is scant with regard to how individuals perceived gender in earlier periods, we do have records of people in various periods who lived all or part of their adult lives in the gender not assigned to them at birth. While these individual cases are often fascinating to contemplate, they must be interpreted cautiously to avoid attributing modern beliefs about gender and sexuality to people from earlier periods. Serious scientific and medical investigation of issues regarding gender and sexual identification dates from the 19th century, and many views on these topics are still evolving.

A BRIEF HISTORICAL OVERVIEW OF GENDER NONCONFORMITY

As Genny Beemyn and Susan Rankin noted in 2014, although gender nonconforming people have existed throughout history, we must remain conscious of the fact that people in past historical times may have had different motivations to dress and/or act as a member of the opposite gender that have nothing to do with our modern notions of gender identity. We must also be aware of the different terminology used to describe behaviors and feeling in different time periods. In the corpus of Google Books, for instance, the term *hermaphrodite* is used with some frequency in the 19th and early 20th centuries, with a peak in the late 19th century, while the term *transsexual* is rarely seen before 1960 and the term *transgender* is rarely seen before 1990. We must also avoid imposing our modern views on the meaning of a specific word or specific behavior on previous time periods.

Even with these reservations, however, it is clear that some people have lived gender nonconforming lives in many different cultures and from ancient times to this day, and this nonconforming behavior has been described in various ways, with various explanations offered, by contemporary and modern historians and theorists. When studying historical cases, it is not always possible to determine which among many possible motivations were paramount in the choice of an individual to live as a member of a sex different than that assigned at birth. The motivation could be personal gender identity, but it could also be related to sexual orientation or the desire to live a life not ordinarily available to one's birth gender, for instance. It could also be related to issues of personal safety or simply the need to earn a living. The latter issue is surprisingly relevant today as well, as a 2006 study by Kristen Schilt and Matthew Wiswall found that male-to-female workers earned about one-third less after their transition, while female-to-male workers actually earned more. Schilt and Wiswall theorize that the difference is due to discrimination against women, so that individuals who transitioned from male to female found themselves paid less due to coworkers and supervisors perceiving them as female, while those who transitioned from female to male were rewarded because they were perceived as men.

Ancient and Classical Greek Philosophy

The term *hermaphrodite* comes from the Greek language and combines the names of Hermes (male) and Aphrodite (female). Several Greek myths discuss the origin of the first hermaphrodite. In one, Hermes and Aphrodite produce a child that they name "Hermaphroditos" since it so perfectly has the attributes of each parent that they are unable to determine if it is a male or a female. In another myth, the child is a male, and falls in love with a female water nymph; the two intertwine their bodies so they become one being, both male and female.

The Greek philosopher Aristotle, who lived in the 4th century BCE, thought that hermaphrodites were a sort of twin, while Galen the Greek/ Roman physician Galen, who lived from approximately CE 129 to CE 200 or 216, believed that hermaphrodites constituted a third sex. The Greek philosopher Plato, who lived from approximately 428 BCE to 348 BCE, discusses the existence of three sexes but says that the hermaphrodite sex disappeared over time, while the male and female sexes persisted.

Some biblical interpreters think that Adam was originally both male and female and only divided into two individuals after falling from grace. The *Tosefta*, a compilation of Jewish oral law probably written in the second or third century CE includes regulations about hermaphrodites (e.g., they could not inherit their father's estates or serve as witnesses or priests), demonstrating that they were recognized as a distinct category of human being.

The United States

The colony of Massachusetts passed a law forbidding cross-dressing in the 1690s, but such laws did not become common in the United States until the mid-19th century. Beginning in the late 1840s, however, many American cities passed laws forbidding individuals from appearing in public in clothing not appropriate to their sex, laws that were probably easier to enforce when there were clearer distinctions made between men's and women's clothing. These laws also reflect the fact that it was more common in the 19th century and earlier when public regulation of individual's dress was more accepted (e.g., some cities had laws forbidding the wearing of clothing associated with a profession or social rank other than one's own). Columbus, Ohio, passed one of the first laws banning cross-dressing, in 1848, and it was only overturned in 1974.

While it is typical to think of transgender people as being clustered in cities, one reason for that impression may be that it is easier for historians to find information about communities of people who acknowledge that they share a common identity than about isolated individuals who may endeavor to hide that same identity. Historian Emily Skidmore, in *True Sex: The Lives of Trans Men at the Turn of the 20th Century*, provides a broader view of the experience of trans men in the United States. Her study, using databases of digitized newspapers from the late 19th and early 20th centuries, was able to demonstrate that many transgender men living in the United States at the turn of the 20th century resided in small towns and successfully "passed" as biologically male for years.

Some Notable Individuals

There's not a lot of information available about transgender people as a group before the mid- to late 20th century, but the stories of some individuals have come down to us. While one should be wary about generalizing from information about specific individuals to larger groups, their life stories are often fascinating and can provide some idea of laws and social customs regarding gender in different historical periods and geographic locations. For instance, in France in 1601, Marie le Marcis, who had lived as a woman for 21 years, decided to begin living as a man, and proceeded to assume the name of Marin and marry a woman. Marin was arrested and threatened with execution, then set free on the condition that he live as Marie and wear women's clothing. Also in 1601, in Italy, a soldier named Daniel Burghammer was revealed to be intersex when he gave birth to a child. Burghammer had been designated male at birth, lived as a man, and was married and had served as a soldier for seven years. Burghammer told his commanding officer that he was both male and female, and eventually the church allowed his wife to divorce him, reasoning that an individual who gave birth could not be a husband.

In 1745 in England, a woman born in Worcester, England, began dressing as a man and using the name James Gray. Her motivation was to search for her husband, a Dutch sailor who had deserted her, and to that end she joined the British navy and passed as a man for five years, returning home after learning that her husband was dead. She became a public sensation after revealing that she was a woman and appeared in stage performances wearing a man's military uniform. "James Gray" continued to dress as a man after retiring, suggesting that the choice to don male garb may have been motivated by more than the opportunity it offered to search for her husband.

Margaret Ann Bulkley was born in the late 19th century in Ireland and was raised as a girl. She later assumed the identity "James Barry," obtained a medical degree, and served as a military surgeon in the British army. As James Barry, she successfully passed as a man her entire adult life and enjoyed a distinguished career, serving in several locations including South Africa and the West Indies; her final position was as inspector general of hospitals in Canada. After retirement in 1859, Barry lived a quiet life in London, and her gender identity was revealed to the public only after her death (contrary to her wishes, which included the stipulation that no examination of her body should be performed before burial).

Herculine Barbin, born in France in 1838, was classified at birth as female and raised as a girl. However, in puberty, she did not develop a female figure nor begin to menstruate, while she did begin to grow facial hair typical of a young man. A physical examination in 1860 revealed that Barbin was probably an intersex individual, with a masculine body type and undescended testicles but the outward genitalia of a woman. A French court declared that she was legally male, and as a result she was forced to change her name and leave her teaching post at a girls' school; in 1868 she committed suicide. Barbin's memoirs, originally published in the 19th century, were discovered by Michel Foucault during his research for his three-volume *History of Sexuality* (published in French 1976–1984, and in English 1978–1986), and his discussion of them brought her life story to a wide audience.

In 1843, only men were allowed to vote in the United States. When Levi Suydam of Connecticut tried to register to vote in 1843, his gender identity was challenged because some felt he was female. A physician examined Suydam and declared that he was in fact male, and he was allowed to vote. However, an additional examination suggest that Suydam may have been intersex, as he had a typically female figure (narrow shoulders, broad hips) and had a vaginal opening through which he menstruated.

Murray Hall was a well-known New York City politician in the last three decades of the 19th century; he served as a member of the General Committee of Tammany Hall and regularly socialized with other male politicians. Hall was married twice (to women) and voted for many years as a man, but after his death in 1901 it was revealed that he had the body of a woman. Later research suggested that Hall was born "Mary Anderson" in Scotland, was orphaned at a young age, and began dressing as a man because that made it easier to find work.

Lili Elbe is among the first individuals known to have had gender reassignment surgery. Because of the destruction of many records during the Nazi period and World War II, there are many questions about her life that remain unanswered, although the broad outlines are known. Born in Denmark in 1882, Elbe was identified as male at birth and given the name Einar Magnus Andreas Wegener. Wegener became a painter and married another painter, Gerda Gottlieb, in 1904. Later, Elbe began to identify as woman and underwent several sex reassignment surgeries in Germany in 1930 and 1931. Such surgeries were highly experimental at the time, and Elbe died of cardiac arrest following a postsurgical infection. Her story has become well known through David Ebershoff's novel *The Danish Girl* and the 2015 film of the same name directed by Tom Hooper.

Christine Jorgenson remains one of the best-known transgender individuals in American history. She was identified as male at birth and served in the U.S. Army during World War II. In the early 1950s, she had transgender surgery in Denmark and the United States and became a celebrity after her story was published in the *New York Daily News* in 1952. Jorgenson worked as an actress and nightclub performer and also gave many public talks in which she discussed her experience.

Unlike Jorgenson, until fairly recently most transgender people chose to conceal their status, instead simply presenting themselves as the gender they identified with or which they perceived to be most advantageous. One such example is Billy Tipton, an American jazz pianist and bandleader who was classified as female at birth and was raised as a girl but took on a male identity as an adult. In his career as a jazz musician, Tipton always presented himself as a man, and eventually adopted a male identity for his private life as well. Tipton avoided medical care in order to conceal his birth gender, and died of an untreated ulcer in 1989; his physical gender identity was revealed to the public not long afterward. Some family members noted that Tipton could not have had the musical career he did if the public had known he was female, so it is unclear if his motivations for taking on a male identity were professional, personal, or both.

As the general public has become more accepting of transgender people, and as laws have been passed to protect their rights, more individuals are publicly identifying as transgender. Examples include journalist Janet Mock, actress Laverne Cox, former Olympic decathlon champion Caitlyn Jenner, film directors Lilly and Lana Wachowski, model Hari Nef, politician Danica Roem, actress Alexis Arquette, retired physician/tennis player Renée Richards, and martial artist Fallon Fox.

Bruce/Brenda/David Reimer

David Reimer deserves particular mention because of the various versions of the life that have been used to serve different arguments about transgender people. His story is well known to the gender public thanks to a 1997 *Rolling Stone* article by John Colapinto, later expanded into a book, *As Nature Made Him: The Boy Who Was Raised as a Girl.* Even before publication of Colapinto's article, Reimer was well known to people in the medical community interested in issues of gender identity, although the version presented in that context was misleading, as will be described next. Reimer's story provides an illustration of the importance of gender identity and the folly of emphasizing the appearance of external genitalia in determining a child's gender; to some people, including many in the trans community, it is also a horror story about a presumptuous medical professional who prioritized his theories and career over the well-being of a patient.

Reimer, born Bruce Peter Reimer in Canada in 1965, was one of a pair of twin boys; his brother was named Brian. (For the sake of clarity, David Reimer will be referred to by that name; other names he was known by will appear inside quotation marks.) Due to an accident during a circumcision when he was seven months old, David's penis was damaged, and his parents were concerned that he would not be able to function normally as a boy and man. They consulted with Dr. John Money, a pediatrician and professor at Johns Hopkins University, who advised them to raise David as a girl. Money believed that gender identity was developed due to social learning, and a case study tracing the maturation of a pair of identical twins, one raised as a boy and one as a girl, offered him an ideal opportunity to test this theory. He also believed that there was a "gender gate" that closed at age two, so that up to that age a child could be assigned to either gender and successfully adapt to the assigned gender, but that successful reassignment was not probable after that point. In Money's reports of this case, David was referred to as "John/Joan."

As a child, David, given the name "Brenda," underwent numerous surgeries, including removal of his testes and creation of a vulva. "Brenda" was also given estrogen during her adolescence, in order to give her a more typically female appearance (e.g., she developed breasts), and Money pressured the family to bring "Brenda" in for surgery to create a vagina. Money acted as "Brenda's" psychologist and published numerous case reports, which supported his theories that even someone who was born biologically male (not intersex) could successfully adjust to life as a female. Money's reports claimed that "Brenda" was happy as a girl, something later contested by David.

Money's account of David's case remained largely unchallenged until the publication of Colapinto's article in 1997. In this article and the subsequent book, based on interviews with David Reimer, all the key points of Money's version were contradicted. David said that he never identified as a girl, hated wearing girls' clothing, and preferred typical "boy" activities like running and climbing over "girl" activities such as playing with dolls. He said that as a child he was ostracized by his peers and was bullied by them as well as by his twin brother and had suffered from depression and suicidal ideation. David also reported that Money had him engage in proto-sexual behaviors with his brother and took sexually suggestive photographs of him. His parents did not tell him about his past, including his gender reassignment, until 1980, when he was 14 years old. At that point, he decided to take the name David and assume a male gender identity. David underwent surgical and hormonal treatments to counteract the effects of the attempts to make him female, and in 1990 married a woman.

Besides the harm done to David Reimer, Money's falsified reports influenced many parents and physicians regarding the kind of care that should be provided to children with ambiguous genitalia. In particular, Money's reports had supported the case for early gender assignment surgery for children born with intersex characteristics, which by definition would need to be performed long before the child's gender identity is known. Reimer's account of his own story, which contradicted Money's version on major points, caused many to reconsider the need or advisability of choosing a gender for a child before the child can have any input into the decision.

SCIENTIFIC AND MEDICAL STUDY OF TRANSGENDER PEOPLE

The historical record prior to the 19th century is scarce regarding scientific and medical study of individuals who did not fit into a conventional male/female dichotomy. In addition, prior to the 19th century, the terms *gender* and *sex* were typically used as synonyms, without consideration of the possibility that a person's gender identity could be different from their sex assigned at birth.

One of the first scientists to contemplate the possibility of intermediate states between male and female was the French zoologist Isidore Geoffroy Saint-Hilaire. Saint-Hilaire, who was elected a member of the French Academy of Sciences in 1833, developed a new science, teratology, focused on classifying unusual births. He argued that even births that might seem monstrous to conventional points of view were part of nature, and that birth anomalies such as hermaphroditism were the result of abnormal embryonic development. Saint-Hilaire believed that studying "abnormal" gender development could help explain normal gender development and illuminate issues such as sexual and gender differences.

Saint-Hilaire believed the body had six "sex segments" or zones, which could be either male or female. In his classification system, there were three segments on either half (left and right) of the body: the profound zone contained ovaries and testicles, the middle zone contained the uterus and seminal vesicles, and the external zone contained external genitalia. If all these zones were in congruence, a body was clearly either male or female, while if some of the zones had male characteristics and some female, the body was a hermaphrodite.

The Scottish obstetrician James Young Simpson built on Saint-Hilaire's system, classifying hermaphrodites as "true" if they had genital organs of both sexes, such as both testes and a uterus, or "spurious" if they had imperfectly developed sex organs of one sex only, even if those organs were similar to those of the opposite sex. The German physician Theodor Albrecht Klebs used a similar system of classification, describing hermaphrodites as "true" if they had both ovarian and testicular tissues, and "pseudo" if they had other sexually identified characteristics of both genders but not both ovarian and testicular tissue. Klebs believed that hermaphrodites were either male or female, as determined by gonadal tissue, no matter how many characteristics of the other sex might be present.

The gonadal definition of hermaphroditism was dominant in the late 19th century, in part because it embraced modern scientific approaches like examining tissue under a microscope. However, it did not allow for considerations of psychology or sociology such as gender roles or gender identity. An 1896 paper by the British physicians George F. Blackler and William P. Lawrence examined a number of claims of hermaphroditism, dismissing all but 3 out of 28 as not meeting modern scientific standards (based on the presence of both male and female gonadal tissue, as determined by microscopic examination).

A different approach was taken by the 19th-century German author and advocate, Karl Friedrich Ulrichs, who was also notable for declaring his homosexuality publicly at a time when homosexual behavior was prohibited by law. Ulrichs recognized the concept of sexual preference and developed a set of terms describing people according to their sexual desires. These terms, which drew on concepts from Plato's *Symposium*, became widely known, particularly *Urning* ("Uranian" in English), which Ulrichs used to describe a man who desired other men. Other terms coined by Ulrichs included *Dioining* for a man who desired women, and *Zwitter* for an intersex person.

The German physician Magnus Hirschfeld was one of the premier sex researchers of the late 19th and early 20th century. He is well known for, among many other things, coining the term *transvestite*, publishing the first scientific study of transvestitism, and publishing the first periodical devoted to the study of sexual minorities, the *Jahrbuch für Sexuelle Zwischenstufen* (*Yearbook for Sexual Intermediates*). Hirschfeld recognized that an individual's gender identity might be different from his or her gender as assigned at birth, and that the desire to dress in clothes of the opposite sex could exist entirely distinct from the desire to engage in sex with others of the same sex. However, while arguing that a transvestite could be of any sexual orientation or sex, he did not distinguish between people who primarily lived as the gender to which they were assigned at birth, but sometimes dressed in clothing of the opposite gender, and those who lived their lives as a gender they were not assigned at birth, for whom wearing clothing associated with that of the opposite gender was an expression of their own gender identification. Hirschfeld argued that *inverts*, a term used at the time to describe men attracted to men and women attracted to women, should be considered a third sex, with members having the opposite characteristics of those believed to be possessed by members of their biological sex. For instance, "normal" women were believed to be passive, but invert women were active and sexual, like men, while male inverts were considered to have "feminine" qualities such as weakness and passivity.

In 1915, the British physician William Blair Bell challenged the primacy of the gonadal system of gender classification, arguing that numerous factors should be considered in determining an individual's gender. For instance, one of his patients had a mix of physical male and female traits, including female breasts, a mustache, a deep voice, an enlarged clitoris. A biopsy revealed that this individual's gonads contained both egg-producing and sperm-producing tissues. Bell concluded that in this case the predominance of female characteristics meant the individual should adopt a female role, as contemporary society would not accept hermaphrodites. At the same time, he believed that the physician should treat each case as an individual, taking into account behavior and all the evidence presented by a particular patient.

For decades, much of the Western understanding of sexuality was taken from the works of Sigmund Freud, a Viennese physician and the creator of psychoanalysis. While Freud's ideas are less embraced today, they are still influential in some quarters. Freud's focus was on the object of desire for an individual, with homosexuals and heterosexuals being defined based on their choice of sexual object (same sex or opposite sex). Freud generally considered homosexuality as a form of arrested development, in which a normal feeling from childhood persisted into adulthood, and offered four different theories for the causes of homosexual desire: the Oedipus conflict and castration anxiety, over-attraction and over-identification with the mother, an inverted Oedipus complex in which the individual takes on a feminine identification to seek the approval of other men, and conversion of the jealousy of the father and other brothers into the love of men.

In 1937, the American physician Hugh Hampton Young published *Genital Abnormalities, Hermaphroditism and Related Adrenal Diseases*, which contained many case histories of intersex people. Notably, Young did not simply describe the bodies of those included in this volume but also discussed their lives and included their own thoughts regarding their bodies. Some of the intersex people he included were quite aware of the societal implications of being one sex or the other, such as the higher earning capacity and personal freedom enjoyed by those classified as male. In the 1940s, American psychologist Albert Ellis studied 84 cases of intersex individuals and concluded that the development of gender and sexuality was based on how an individual was socialized as well as the biological makeup of their body.

In the late 1940s and early 1950s, the term *transsexual* began to be used more commonly for people who identified with a gender not congruent with that to which they had been assigned at birth. Harry Benjamin, an American endocrinologist, was among the first to recognize that a person's sense of gender identity seemed to persist despite attempts to change it by psychotherapy and argued that people whose gender identity did not match their bodies should be allowed to use hormones and surgery to bring the two into congruence. Benjamin also noted that gender nonconformity existed on a spectrum, while the clinical approach to transgender people in this period focused on identifying people who wanted to make a complete change from male to female or female to male.

In the 1970s, Sandra Bem created the *Bem Sex-Role Inventory*, a self-report instrument allowing individuals to describe themselves on a number of characteristics considered typically masculine or feminine in American culture at the time. Bem's inventory acknowledged that an individual's identity as masculine or feminine could be placed on a continuum and was not necessarily congruent with their sex as assigned at birth. Her research helped highlight traits and characteristics considered appropriate for one sex or the others by societal conventions and helped to separate two distinct concepts: an individual's dissatisfaction with societal expectations and role assignment based on their birth sex, and an individual's perception that their gender does not correspond with their assigned sex.

Although the work of Alfred Kinsey, including his groundbreaking reports *Sexual Behavior in the Human Male* (1948) and *Sexual Behavior in the Human Female* (1953) did not specifically focus on transgender individuals, his concept of classifying sexual behavior on a spectrum rather than a dichotomy contributed to challenging assumptions about gender and sexuality. Kinsey believed that many people are not exclusively gay or straight, but may engage in sex with both members of the opposite sex and members of their own sex, and developed a scale ranging from 0 (exclusively heterosexual) to 6 (exclusively homosexual) to describe individuals; he also included an eighth category, X, for individuals without sexual contacts or reactions.

TRANSGENDER PEOPLE AND THE *DSM*

The *Diagnostic and Statistical Manual of Mental Disorders* or *DSM*, published by the American Psychiatric Association (APA), is commonly regarded as the most authoritative professional source for information about mental and psychiatric illness. The attempt to create a classification of mental disorders dates back to ancient times, but the need for an accepted set of categories increased in the 19th and early 20th centuries due to the interest in collecting statistical data relating to mental health. For instance, by the late 19th century, seven categories of mental illness were recognized in the United States—mania, melancholia, monomania, paresis, dementia, dipsomania, and epilepsy. Following several other efforts to create a categorization system for mental illness, the first edition of the *DSM* was published in 1952; it drew heavily on the sixth edition of the *International Classification of Diseases* (*ICD-6*) published by the World Health Organization and on a classification system developed by the Veterans Administration. Various innovations were included in later editions—for instance the *DSM-III*, published in 1980, was the first to include explicit diagnostic criteria and drew heavily on validation research that examined the usefulness of those criteria.

Of course, the *DSM* is created by human beings and reflects general societal attitudes as well as those of the psychiatric profession, both facts that influence what is or is not considered a disease or disorder. Because it is regarded as authoritative and is used in the training and practice of people who work in the field of mental illness (including psychologists and social workers as well as psychiatrists), the choices made in the *DSM* matter to individuals outside those professions as well. For instance, for years homosexuality was classified as a mental disorder, a fact used to justify "treatments" such as aversion therapy to attempt to "cure" a gay person of his or her sexual preference. Due in part to the growing gay rights movement, many people felt this classification stigmatized a normal human state of being rather than a disease to be cured. In 1973, APA members voted at their annual convention to remove homosexuality from the *DSM*, while adding the category "sexual orientation disturbance." Crucially, "sexual orientation disturbance" applied only to those who experienced conflict due to their sexual orientation, rather than those who simply had a sexual orientation other than heterosexual.

In 1980, the third edition of the *DSM* (*DSM-III*) included, for the first time, diagnoses for gender identity disorder for children and transsexualism for adults. The terminology used to refer to gender identity continued to evolve, and in the revised version of the third edition, (*DSM III-R*), published in 1987, the diagnosis of gender identity disorder of adolescence and adulthood, nontranssexual type was added. In the fourth edition (*DSM-IV*), published in 1994, all three conditions were included under one diagnosis, gender identity disorder, with separate diagnostic criteria provided for children and adults. The most recent edition (*DSM-5*, published in 2013) replaces the term *gender identity disorder* with *gender dysphoria*, and provides one set of diagnostic criteria for children and another for adolescents and adults.

There are positive aspects to the inclusion of these categories within the *DSM*: for instance, insurance companies often use inclusion in the *DSM* as a criterion for authorizing treatment, and thus transgender people are better able to access and pay for their care. On the other hand, inclusion in the *DSM* may support the argument that an individual's gender identity, or their way of suppressing it, is a problem that should be corrected rather than simply their way of existing in the world. Perhaps recognizing this contradiction, the APA issued a fact sheet on gender dysphoria prior to the release of *DSM-5*, stating that gender nonconformity is not a disorder in and of itself, and that a diagnosis of gender dysphoria requires that the individual experience significant distress as a result of the condition (the term *dysphoria* in ordinary language refers to a state of distress or dissatisfaction).

OTHER RESEARCH

Professional social science research on transgender people, or for that matter on minority sexuality people (gay, lesbian, bisexual, etc.) in general, has a relatively short history. Prior to the work of Dr. Evelyn Hooker in the 1950s, much of the research characterizing homosexual men was conducted on psychiatric patients or incarcerated individuals, who were not representative of the gay population as a whole. In retrospect, this seems astonishing (imagine how silly it would seem today if research into heterosexuality were only conducted with prisoners and psychiatric patients!), but it was an accepted practice at the time, and reinforced the prevailing theory that homosexuality was a disorder rather than a normal state of being.

Hooker, an American psychologist who was familiar with discrimination due to her experiences as a woman in academia as well as time spent in Germany as the Nazis were coming to power, received a grant from the National Institute of Mental Health in 1953 to compare gay and straight men on a number of psychological measures. Her gay subjects were recruited with the aid of the Mattachine Society, an early gay rights organization, and each gay man was matched with a straight man on the basis of age, IQ score, and education. Her study revealed that there were no important differences in terms of general adjustment between the gay and straight individuals studied, with about two-thirds of both groups having average or better adjustment. She also demonstrated that other experts who evaluated the test results "blind" (without knowing which group each individual belong to) were unable to determine which individuals were gay and which were straight.

Later research often focused less on the fact that sexual minorities exist, and more on studying how such individuals live. Such research turned over many stereotypes, including that persons of nonstandard sexuality inevitably led lonely and unhappy lives, and that nonstandard sexuality was for many simply a phase that they moved through on the way to adult heterosexuality. Research also documented the actual many ways that people formed relationships and families outside the standard pattern of a married man and woman and their biological children.

In the 21st century, research on transgender people has become a growing field of study, with many different lines of approach. One is on the social service needs of transgender people, and how being a member of a minority sexuality affects their lives. Balancing that recognition is the need to be aware of the diversity among transgender people and the many factors (e.g., race, gender, economic status, educational status) that also influence their lives. Even within these demographic categories, there is variety: just as it should be obvious that not all white heterosexuals, for example, experience the world in the same way, and the same is true for white transgender people, black transgender people, and so on.

Increasing scholarly interest in the transgender community is evident in the number of professional articles published concerning transgender people. One way to take a broad look at trends over the years is to compare the results of searches for articles published in different time periods that use specific terms such as *transgender*. A search of the Academic Search Elite database published by EBSCO, limited to articles in peer-reviewed journals in English, found 37 articles that included either the term *transgender* or *transsexual* published between 1971 and 1980 and 36 such articles published between 1981 and 1990. In contrast, 260 articles containing those terms and published between 1991 and 2000 are included in this database, as are 2,271 published between 2001 and 2010.

CHAPTER 3

Transitioning

Some transgender people go through a process called transitioning or gender transitioning, during which they change either or both of their gender presentation and physical sexual characteristics to match their internal sense of gender. Some people prefer the term *gender affirming transitioning* because it reflects the idea that a person undergoing the process is becoming outwardly who they already knew they were internally. There is no template for transitioning and it is not necessary for a transgender person to go through any formal process to be considered transgender—instead, it is a highly individual experience that is chosen by some transgender person, based on their own desires. Gender transition may involve hormone therapy or surgery, but neither is a requirement, and it may also include other processes such as voice therapy and counseling. This chapter will concentrate on formal aspects of the transitioning process, particularly those that require consultation with medical professionals, but that should not be taken to imply that these processes are the most important in transitioning. An individual can transition without any involvement with a medical professional, and for some individuals, behavioral changes such as (for a transgender man) packing and binding may play a greater role in the transition process than anything else he may choose to do.

GUIDELINES FOR THE GENDER TRANSITION PROCESS

Guidelines issued by the Center of Excellence for Transgender Health of the Department of Family & Community Medicine, University of California, San Francisco, divide the types of gender-affirming interventions typically sought by transgender and gender nonbinary people into three categories: medical interventions (primarily hormone therapy), surgical interventions, and other interventions (such as facial hair removal, speech therapy, genital packing or tucking, and chest binding). Besides providing detailed information for medical professionals guiding individuals through gender transition, the guidelines also evaluate the strength of evidence to evaluate the risks and benefits of specific drugs and treatment regimens.

A transgender individual may desire any combination of these interventions, or no interventions at all. Some may want one or more interventions (e.g., hormone therapy) for a limited period of time, while others may continue the same therapy for a lifetime. For ease of communication, the term *transitioning* is used in this chapter, but that does not imply that anyone seeking one or more of the interventions described here necessarily regards themselves as going through a gender transition. Gender transition is a highly individual process and the best policy for medical and psychological professionals assisting in the process is to treat each case as unique. The guidelines also note that while in the past there was a generally accepted pathway for gender transition (first psychological assessment, then hormone treatment, then surgery), today each transgender person should be allowed to choose exactly what interventions they feel will meet their needs, and in the order they find suits them best.

Medical Interventions

The most common medical intervention for transgender people is hormone therapy. In the past, it was common for a physician to require a patient to present a letter from a mental health professional before the physician would begin to treat the patient with hormone therapy, but today many physicians recognize an "informed consent" path as well. In this latter path, physician evaluates the patient's gender dysphoria and judges if the patient is able to provide informed consent for hormone treatment; such consent would require that the patient understands the risks and benefits of the treatment, is aware of alternatives, and understands the limitations of the treatment. Some changes due to hormone therapy are reversible, while others are permanent, and anyone contemplating hormone therapy should be very clear on which is which before beginning treatment.

Feminizing hormone therapy is used by transgender women to suppress male secondary sex characteristics and develop female secondary sex characteristics. It is usually provided by combining an estrogen with an androgen blocker, and possibly a progestogen as well. Many bodily changes can result from feminizing hormone therapy, including changes in the skin (drier and thinner), breast development, fat redistribution (more on the hips and thighs, more fat just beneath the skin), loss of muscle tissue and strength, reduction in body hair, changes in sweat patterns, and reduced testicular size. Emotional changes often accompany feminizing hormone therapy, as do changes in the libido and in erectile function.

The prescribing physician will also monitor hormone levels and physiological changes in the patient, adjusting dosages as necessary. While the drugs used in feminizing hormone therapy are commonly used in other types of medicine as well, for many there is little scientific data to guide their use in the transgender population. Prescribing feminizing hormones is also complicated because many of the drugs exist in multiple forms (tablet, gel, patch, etc.), and not all forms may be available at the pharmacy used by an individual patient.

Masculinizing hormone therapy is used by transgender men to minimize or suppress female secondary sexual characteristics and develop male secondary sex characteristics. Parenteral (administered by a route other than the mouth, e.g., through a skin patch, a gel, or by injection) testosterone preparations are often used for masculinizing hormone therapy. As with feminizing hormones, although the same drugs are often used in medicine (e.g., to treat cisgender men who have low levels of testosterone), limited data is available to help guide dosages in transgender men.

Effects commonly seen with masculinizing hormones include lowering of voice, changes in the skin (thicker, more oily, possibly resulting in acne), redistribution of body fat and muscle (less fat around the hips and thighs, greater muscular definition), development of facial hair, increased muscle, changes in sweat patterns and body odor, and growth of the clitoris. Some individuals gain weight after starting testosterone therapy, while others lose weight. Some individuals will notice emotional changes, although the stereotypical "'roid rage" (steroid rage) is not the only possibility, and some people report feeling calmer after beginning testosterone therapy. Increased libido (sex drive) is also commonly reported among transgender men taking testosterone. Menstrual periods usually cease, and transmen may experience vaginal dryness as well.

Surgical Interventions

Some transgender people may have one or more surgeries during their transition, while others may never have surgery. People outside the transgender community may hold many misconceptions about the relationship between a person's gender identity and the state of their body. For instance, it is not uncommon for a cisgender person to conceive of the transition process as necessarily culminating in surgery, or believe that a person is not "really" transgender if they haven't had surgery (and typically what is meant is "bottom" surgery on the genitals). This is an ill-informed opinion that should not be supported, and those transgender people who are sufficiently confident and patient may choose to educate others about these misconceptions. Transgender people may also find themselves asked oddly specific questions about their body parts or their preference in sexual activities, but such questions reveal an ignorance of the complexity of gender identity and the very individual nature of the transition process.

A number of surgical interventions are available for persons undergoing gender transition, and the decision as to which are appropriate for the identity of a particular individual can only be determined by that person, with medical advice provided by the physician.

Top surgery refers to surgery on the chest, and many transgender men get top surgery to remove breast tissue and create a more male-looking chest. Top surgery has the advantages of having an immediate and obvious impact on a person's appearance, and is generally less expensive than many "bottom" surgeries. Several different procedures are possible, including double mastectomy with nipple graphing and the keyhole procedure. Breast augmentation, an option chosen by some transgender women, involves increasing the size of the breasts through the use of saline or silicone implants. However, because feminizing hormone use alone will increase breast size, individuals often choose to wait 24 months after beginning feminizing hormones before deciding if they want breast augmentation surgery.

Bottom surgery refers to surgery on the genitals or internal reproductive organs. These surgeries are generally more complex and expensive than top surgery, but for some individuals bottom surgery is exactly what they need to reflect their gender identity. In an orchiectomy, the testicles are removed. Penectomy, or removal of the penis, is also possible but is an operation rarely performed in the United States. Metoidioplasty is a procedure to increase the length of the clitoris by freeing it from the suspensory ligament and from its attachment to the labia minor; this surgery may also include a "urethral hookup" which allows the individual to urinate through a surgically constructed penis. Hysterectomy is removal of the uterus; if the fallopian tubes and ovaries are removed as well, the operation is called a hysterosalpingo-oophorectomy.

Vaginoplasty is the creation of a vagina, often incorporating tissues from the shaft of the penis; often clitoroplasty (creation of a clitoris) using the glans of the penis and labiaplasty (creation of a labia) using scrotal tissue are performed at the same time. Vaginoplasty is a more involved surgery than many other procedures discussed here and may require staying in the hospital for one or more days, as well as a recovery process that can last several months. Phalloplasty, the creation of a penis, is rarely performed in the United States due to high cost and mixed results but may be available in other countries. Scrotoplasty, the creation of a scrotum, involves inserting silicone implants into the labia, possibly following a skin expansion process that can last several months.

Several types of surgery may be performed on the face and neck as part of the transition process. Transgender women sometimes opt for facial feminization surgery (FFS), the term applied to a variety of plastic surgery techniques intended to make an individual look more feminine, such as reshaping the jaw and chin. Transgender women may also opt for a tracheal shave to reduce the size of their Adam's apple, and those with balding or thinning hair may opt for hair transplantation (moving hair follicles from the side and back of the head to the balding areas).

Fertility Considerations

Transgender status does not preclude the desire to have children, and thus any physician providing medical care to or counseling people considering gender transition should advise their patients as to the likely effects of any treatment or procedure on fertility. There are ways to preserve sperm and eggs, which may allow the conception of children after an individual's gonads (testes or ovaries) are removed. For those who opt for hormone therapy but not gonadectomy, fertility may cease while the individual is taking the hormones but be restored after a period (some evidence suggests three to six months) of not taking hormones. On the other hand, hormone therapy alone is not a reliable form of birth control, so some other form of contraception should be used. Because the use of testosterone is associated with birth defects, a trans man who desires to become pregnant should cease using testosterone for some months before attempting to become pregnant; unfortunately, there is not sufficient scientific data to specify exactly how long that period should last.

Fertility preservation methods used with cisgender patients, such as cryopreservation of eggs, sperm, or ovarian or testicular tissue, may also be useful to transgender patients. In addition, transgender patients may want to use assisted reproduction techniques also used by infertile cisgender individuals, such as in vitro fertilization (IVF). IVF may use sperm or eggs from donors and may involve a surrogate or gestational carrier (a woman who carries the pregnancy to term).

Options for Nonbinary Individuals

Some individuals reject the conventional binary of male and female and may describe themselves by terms such as *nonbinary, genderqueer, gender fluid*, or *gender nonconforming*. A nonbinary individual should discuss in detail with his or her medical provider exactly what they need to affirm their identity, including the specific mix of secondary sexual characteristics they desire. For medical interventions, a variety of strategies are available, including using low-dose hormones, using only a subset of the usual hormones prescribed (e.g., using an androgen blocker but not estrogen), and using hormones for a limited amount of time only. A similar decision-making process can guide the nonbinary individual and his or her medical caregiver when considering gender-affirming surgery and honoring the individual's specific desire should be the guiding principle.

HEALTH CONSIDERATIONS DURING AND AFTER TRANSITION

Observational studies have demonstrated that biological sex is associated with a higher probability of certain medical conditions; for instance, men are more likely than women to have cardiovascular disease. However, such studies do not demonstrate that male or female hormones are the reason for the observed differences, because men and women differ in many ways besides their hormonal makeup. For this reason, it is incorrect to jump to the conclusion that, for instance, a transgender man taking testosterone will have an elevated risk of cardiovascular disease compared to a transgender man not on hormone therapy. Another difficulty in advising transgender people about health risks during transition is that relatively few studies have been conducted that could help answer such questions, and some of those that exist have major shortcomings that make it difficult to draw conclusions from them.

Several studies suggest that transgender men taking testosterone do not have an elevated risk for cardiovascular disease, compared to cisgender women. Other studies have indicated that transgender women do have an increased risk for cardiovascular disease as compared to cisgender men, although the largest of these studies, conducted with over 1,000 Dutch transgender and women, did not control for tobacco use, obesity or diabetes, all of which are associated with increased risk of mortality. Although it is difficult to draw conclusions based on the available evidence regarding cardiovascular risk, one option for physicians treating transgender patients is to emphasize behavioral changes that reduce risk, such as weight loss, increased physical activity, smoking cessation, and appropriate management of diabetes.

Diabetes is a common and serious disease—according to the American Diabetes Association, 30 million Americans in 2015 had diabetes (9.4% of the population), and it is the seventh leading cause of death in the United States. Evidence is inconclusive on whether there is increased risk of diabetes for transgender people, but at a minimum they should receive the same screening for diabetes as any patient. Because diabetes may complicate surgery (e.g., greater risk of infection), aggressive measures should be used to normalize glucose control for individuals seeking gender-affirming surgery.

Osteoporosis, a disease in which the bones become weak and brittle and thus more likely to break, is more common in women than men, particularly in women after menopause. However, the United States has no national guidelines for screening patients for osteoporosis, which complicates the effort to make recommendations for screening transgender patients. Studies of bone density in transgender women following hormone treatment have produced equivocal results, so it is not possible to associate the use of feminizing hormones with increased osteoporosis risk. However, some studies have found that the male-to-female transition is associated with other factors, such as reduced physical activity levels and lower levels of vitamin D, that are associated with osteoporosis, so this should be kept in mind. Most studies of transgender men find increased bone density, or no change, following hormone therapy.

Guidelines for HIV screening and care are the same for transgender individuals as for the general public, although care providers should be aware of the high rates of trauma and intersecting patterns of discrimination faced by many transgender people, particularly transgender women. Transgender men generally have a lower rate of HIV infection than transgender women, although there is evidence that HIV rates are increasing among transgender men who have sex with men. Risk assessment may also be complicated for transgender patients, and the physician must have sufficient trust from the patient to obtain accurate information about exactly what sexual activities the patient engages in. Besides condoms (including female condoms for individuals who engage in receptive vaginal sex), physicians should ensure that patients are aware of the options of pre-exposure prophylaxis (PrEP) and nonoccupational post-exposure prophylaxis (nPEP).

There is not sufficient data to determine if cancer risk changes due to hormone treatment. Individuals should be screened for cancer according to the body organs they have—for instance, if a transgender man has a cervix, he is still at risk for cervical cancer and should be screened for it.

TRANSITION STORIES

Transitioning is a highly individual process and may involve major changes to the transitioning individual's body. While appropriate medical and psychological guidance should be sought as relevant during the process, many individuals find useful information about the process from reading the stories of others. Fortunately, many individuals today have chosen to come forward with their gender transition stories, and learning about their experiences may help others to understand what their options are and what aspects of the transition process will be most useful for them. One source of information is the Internet—a search on terms like *stories of gender transition* will turn up many articles as well as entire websites devoted to this topic. Another source of information are books and movies, and a similar search will turn up many autobiographies in book and movie form that may serve useful.

DETRANSITIONING

Detransitioning refers to the process of reversing some or all of a gender transition. It is impossible to state how many transgender people have detransitioned (indeed, it's not possible to state with any authority how many transgender people exist at all, or how many have gone through what aspects of gender transition), but the subject has received some coverage in the news media. Some of this coverage has been of an exploitative nature, sometimes in the guise of "raising the question" of how much money was being spent on such individuals and suggesting that it was wasted. While it's true that some transgender people do detransition, the subject is not a simple one and should be approached with a respect for the individuals involved and their particular circumstances and choices. The fact that some people do detransition, in part or in whole, temporarily or permanently, should not be used to question whether transgender people actually exist or whether the transition problem itself is valid.

There is limited scientific study of those who detransition; for instance, one 50-year-old study from Sweden did not directly address detransitioning but found that 2.2 percent of people who underwent medical gender transition later experienced regret about having done so. It's worth noting that this is much lower than the proportion of people who report that they regret having plastic surgery on their nose, a proportion that has been esti-mated at 17 percent. In addition, the individual cases of detransitioning reported in the popular press should not be used to draw conclusion about the transgender population as a whole, because we simply don't have enough information yet to understand who detransitions, why, and how the detransition process affects the lives of those who choose that path.

Eight percent of respondents to the 2015 National Transition Sur-vey reported detransitioning at some point, that is, returning to living as the gender they were assigned at birth; however, most detransitioned only temporarily, and 62 percent of those who had once detransitioned reported currently living in their felt gender identity. Detransitioning was more common among transgender women (11%) than transgender men (4%). Comparing racial and ethnic groups, detransitioning was most com-mon among American Indians (14%), followed by Asians and multiracial individuals (10% each), Hispanics (9%), blacks and whites (8% each), and was least common among Middle Eastern individuals (5%). Among those who detransitioned, the most common reasons given included pres-sure from a parent (36%), transitioning was too difficult (33%), discrimi-nation and harassment as a transgender person (31%), trouble getting a job (29%), pressure from other family members (not a spouse or parent) (26%), pressure from a spouse or partner (18%), and pressure from an employer (17%).

Just as every transgender person is unique, so is every person who chooses to detransition. A variety of motivations have been cited by those who have made this choice. Some are concerned about the effects of hor-mones on their health, or do not wish to give up their fertility due to either surgery or hormone treatment. Some are uncomfortable with their new role, and in the case of males who transition to female, regret the loss of status, loss of income, and newfound experiences of gender-based dis-crimination and harassment as they become publicly perceived as women. Some individuals may have had unrealistic expectations for the transition process (as some do for, say, plastic surgery on their nose or breasts, as if their changed physical appearance would be some kind of magic cure for all their problems). Some may also discover, after completing the transi-tion, that neither gender appropriately defines them, and they are happier with a nonbinary or identity; in that case, they may not feel the need to continue taking hormones or proceeding with other aspects of the transi-tion process.

People need medical, psychological, and social support during the transition process, and this is even more the case if they are experiencing difficulty with their new identity. Unfortunately, there are few guidelines for helping people who are considering detransitioning, and they may find it even more difficult than those undergoing gender transition to get appropriate help and advice. Besides professional care and advice, information is available from other people who are considering detransition or have gone through the detransition process, which can be accessed on websites such as Detransition Info or by searching the Internet for terms such as *detransition story.*

CHAPTER 4

Physical Health

Everyone is concerned with their health, and transgender people are no exception. In addition to general health issues, transgender people face specific concerns related to their trans status, beginning with whether health insurance will cover procedures related to transitioning. There are a whole host of questions about what, if any, surgical or hormonal treatment is appropriate in childhood for children born with nonconforming genitals, or whose other sexual characteristics do not conform to the standard male/female dichotomy. And although everyone should be concerned about HIV and other sexually transmitted diseases, trans people are at particular risk, and that risk is particularly high for trans people in some demographics. Trans people also face issues in terms of patient–provider relations and health insurance coverage, the latter of particular significance in the United States as we do not have a national health system.

GENERAL HEALTH

United States

According to data from the 2015 U.S. Transgender Survey, overall the health of transgender individuals is similar to that of the U.S. population as a whole. One commonly used measure of general health is asking respondents to describe their current state of health on a five-point scale: Excellent, Very Good, Good, Fair, or Poor. Respondents to the Transgender Survey rated their general health as follows: 12 percent excellent, 33 percent very good, 33 percent good, 17 percent fair, and 5 percent poor. This pattern is similar to that of the general U.S. population for the same year, as measured by the Behavioral Risk Factor Surveillance System, on which 19 percent report being in excellent health, 32 percent very good health, 32 percent good health, 13 percent fair health, and 5 percent good health.

There was variance within the transgender respondents, however, related to factors including gender identity, age, and family support. While overall 45 percent of the transgender sample reported being in excellent or very good health, only 35 percent of nonbinary individuals designated female on their original birth certificate reported being in excellent or very good health. In contrast, 47 percent of transgender men, 50 percent of transgender women, 57 percent of cross-dressers, and 50 percent of nonbinary individuals designated as male on their original birth certificates reported being in excellent or very good health. In the transgender sample, older age groups tended to report better overall health, which is the opposite of the trend usually observed in the general population (in which older age is associated with worse general health). The highest percentage reporting excellent or very good health in the transgender sample was those age 65 or over (60%), followed by those age 45 through 64 (53%), those age 25 through 44 (48%), and those age 18 through 24 (39%). Individuals who describe their family as supportive were more likely to report being in excellent or very good health (52%) as compared to those who describe their family support as neutral (42%) or unsupportive (38%).

Canada

The Canadian Trans Youth Health Study asked respondents (age 14–25) to rate their health status on a five-point scale: Excellent, Very Good, Good, Fair, Poor. Most youths (41%) rated their health as good, with 30 percent indicating their health was fair, 16 percent very good, 9 percent poor, and 4 percent excellent. This is somewhat lower than might be expected from a young sample—for instance, on the 2001–2002 National Health and Nutrition Examination Survey conducted in the United States, among adolescents age 12–15 years, 63 percent indicated that their health was excellent or very good.

TRANSITION-RELATED CARE

The respondents of the 2015 National Transgender Survey indicated significant levels of unmet needs with regard to transition-related health care. For instance, 78 percent desired hormone therapy at some point, but only 49 percent had received it. Transgender men and women were both more likely to want hormone therapy (95%) and to receive it (71%), as compared to nonbinary respondents, of whom 49 percent wanted hormone therapy and 13 percent received it. Higher income was strongly associated with receiving hormone therapy; among people reporting no income, only 31 percent had received hormone therapy, as compared to 37 percent with incomes between $1 and $9,999, 55 percent of those with incomes between $10,000 and $24,000, 64 percent of those with incomes between $25,000 and $49,000, 66 percent of those with incomes between $50,000 and $99,000, and 64 percent of those with incomes of $100,000 or more.

Most of the respondents who had received hormone therapy began receiving it between the ages of 18 and 24 (41%) or 25 to 44 (43%), with 4 percent beginning hormone therapy before age 18 and 13 percent after age 45. Most (91%) who received hormone therapy reported receiving their hormones from licensed professionals only, but 6 percent said they received them from both licensed professionals and friends, and 2 percent only from non-licensed sources such as friends or online sources. However, those without health insurance were more likely to receive hormones from non-licensed sources only (10%), as were those currently involved in the underground economy (e.g., drug sales, sex work) (8%), who had done sex work at some point in their lives (5%), or who were living in poverty (4%). Fifteen percent of respondents said that they had wanted to use puberty-blocking medications (hormone suppressors that can delay the physical changes of puberty), but fewer than 1 percent actually received these medications.

One-quarter (25%) of respondents had received some type of surgery related to their transition, with surgery more common among transgender men (42%) and among transgender women (28%) or nonbinary individuals (9%). Higher income was associated with a higher probability of transgender surgery: only 12 percent of those who reported no income had received any transgender surgery, as compared to 15 percent of those with incomes between $1 and $9,999, 24 percent of those with incomes between $10,000 and $24,000, 36 percent of those with incomes between $25,000 and $49,000, 43 percent of those with incomes between $50,000 and $99,000, and 43 percent of those with incomes of $100,000 or more. Type of insurance was also related to receiving transition-related surgery: 44 percent of those on Medicare only reported receiving surgery for gender transition, as compared to 32 percent with multiple insurance types, 25 percent with private insurance only, 22 percent each for those with Medicaid only or other insurance only, and 18 percent for those with no insurance.

Among those designated as female on their original birth certificate, 21 percent had had chest reduction or reconstruction, 8 percent a hysterectomy, 1 percent metoidioplasty, and 1 percent phalloplasty. An additional 52 percent indicated that they wanted to have chest reduction or reconstruction in the future, 44 percent wanted a hysterectomy in the future, 15 percent wanted metoidioplasty in the future, and 11 percent wanted phalloplasty in the future. Transgender men were more likely to have had, and to want to have, these procedures, as compared to nonbinary individuals—for instance, 97 percent of transgender men had either had chest reduction or reconstruction surgery, while only 48 percent of nonbinary individuals had either had or desired such surgery.

Among those designated as male on their original birth certificate, by far the most common procedure was hair removal or electrolysis: 41 percent had had this procedure, and an additional 49 percent indicated that they wanted to have it in the future. In addition, 11 percent said they had had nonsurgical voice therapy and an additional 46 percent wanted to have it in the future, 10 percent had had vaginoplasty or labiaplasty and 45 percent wanted to have it in the future, 9 percent had had orchiectomy and 40 percent wanted to have it in the future, 8 percent had had augmentation mammoplasty and 36 percent wanted to have it in the future, 6 percent had had facial feminization surgery and 39 percent wanted to have it in the future, 4 percent had had a tracheal shave and 29 percent wanted to have it in the future, 2 percent had received silicone injection and 9 percent wanted to receive them in the future, and 1 percent had had voice surgery and 16 percent wanted to have it in the future. Transgender women were more likely than nonbinary individuals to have had these procedures or to desire to have them some day—for instance, 95 percent of transgender women had or wanted to have hair removal or electrolysis, as compared to 67 percent of nonbinary individuals.

HEALTH ISSUES RELATED TO HORMONE THERAPY

Standards of Care for the Health of Transsexual, Transgender, and Gender Nonconforming People includes a review of research related to medical complications of hormone therapy, based on several literature reviews and one large study. These risks are listed separately for feminizing (i.e., used in male-to-female transition) and masculinizing (used in female-to-male transition) hormone therapy and are classified as "likely increased risk," "possible increased risk," and "inconclusive or no increased risk," based on the strength of evidence in each case.

For feminizing hormone therapy, there are four categories of likely increased risk: venous thromboembolic disease, cardiovascular and cerebrovascular disease (disease of the heart and blood vessels, and of the blood vessels supplying the brain), lipids (fats, including cholesterol and triglycerides), and liver and gallbladder. Estrogen use increases the risk of venous thrombolic events (VTE, a blood clot in a vein), with increased risk for those who are over age 40, smoke, are sedentary, obese, have underlying thrombophilic disorders (disorders that increase the likelihood of clots forming in the blood), or who use third generation progestins. The risk is decreased if estradiol (a form of estrogen) is delivered transdermally (through a skin patch), and this mode of delivery is recommended for patients with an increased risk of VTE. For patients over age 50 with underlying cardiovascular risk factors, estrogen use increases the risk of cardiovascular events, and this risk may be increased if additional progestin is used. The use of oral estrogen is associated with increased triglycerides, which increases the risk of cardiovascular and pancreatic disease, and the use of transdermal estrogen is recommended for patients with preexisting lipid disorders. Estrogen use increases the risk of gall stones (cholelithiasis) and for the need to surgically remove the gallbladder (cholecystectomy), and the use of estrogen and cyproterone acetate may be associated with transient elevation of liver enzymes and more rarely with clinical hepatotoxicity (damage to the liver).

The use of feminizing hormones carries three types of possible increased risk: for type 2 diabetes mellitus (diabetes characterized by insulin resistance), hypertension (high blood pressure), and prolactinoma (overproduction of the hormone prolactin by the pituitary gland). Increased risk of type 2 diabetes is particularly associated with the use of estrogen and among patients with other risks factors (including family history of diabetes) for this disease. Estrogen may increase blood pressure, although the risk for overt hypertension (blood pressure over 140/90 Hg) is unknown. The risk for hypertensive patients or those at high risk for hypertension maybe is lowered through the use of the diuretic spironolactone. The risk of prolactinoma may be increased with estrogen use in the first year of treatment but is unlikely after this period, and estrogen use may raise preexisting prolactinoma to levels high enough to trigger a clinical diagnosis.

For breast cancer, the evidence is not sufficient to draw a conclusion about whether feminizing hormones increase risk. Transwomen can develop breast cancer, but there is insufficient evidence to compare their risk to that of cisgender women. It is likely that long-term use of feminizing estrogen, the use of progestins, and other risk factors such as obesity and family history of breast cancer is associated with increased breast cancer risk (as is the case with cisgender women), but the evidence is insufficient to draw a firm conclusion. There are several other changes associated with the use of feminizing hormones, which a patient may consider negative, minor, or positive. These include a drop in fertility, decreased libido (sexual desire), and a reduction in nocturnal emissions ("wet dreams").

Some individuals take antiandrogen medications, also known as testosterone blockers or androgen antagonists, to inhibit the production or effects of testosterone. Spironolactone is a diuretic that is also used as an antiandrogen medication; known side effects, based on its use in treating hypertension and congestive heart failure, include dizziness, gastrointestinal symptoms (e.g., stomach irritation), and hyperkalemia (high levels of potassium in the blood stream). Cyproterone acetate, a progestogen with antiandrogenic properties that is not approved for use in the United States but is available in some other countries (e.g., it is used in the United Kingdom to treat prostate cancer). It is associated with a number of side effects, including, rarely, hepatotoxicity (liver damage).

Research has identified two likely increased risks associated with the use of masculinizing therapy. The use of testosterone or other androgenic steroids is associated with an increased risk for polycythemia (increased hemoglobin in the blood). This risk is increased for patients with other risk factors and may be decreased if the drug is delivered transdermally (via a skin path) and a change in dosage may also decrease the risk. Masculinizing hormone therapy is also associated with weight gain and an increase in visceral fat (fat stored in the abdominal cavity).

Masculinizing therapy is associated with possible increased risk of several conditions. Lipids may be affected, usually with a decrease in HDL ("good cholesterol") and variable effects on LDL ("bad cholesterol") and triglycerides. Transdermal administration is less likely to cause these effects than intramuscular use (injections), particularly when the latter is used to raise serum levels of cholesterol beyond the normal male range. Testosterone therapy may temporarily raise the level of liver enzymes, and the use of oral methyltestosterone has been associated with negative effects to the liver. Psychiatric symptoms may increase in patients with underlying psychiatric disorders who are taking masculinizing hormones, including increased hypomanic, manic, and psychotic symptoms; these effects are most associated with high doses of hormones.

For a number of other conditions, there is insufficient evidence to conclude if the use of masculinizing hormones results in increased risk. These conditions include osteoporosis, cardiovascular events and disease, hypertension, type 2 diabetes mellitus, breast cancer, cervical cancer, ovarian cancer, and endometrial cancer (cancer of the layer of cells lining the uterus). Other side effects of masculinizing therapy, which may be considered undesirable, desirable, or minor, depending on the patient, included reduction in fertility, changes in a developing embryo or fetus, enlargement of the clitoris, increased libido, acne, and male pattern hair loss.

SURGERY ON INTERSEX CHILDREN

While it is not possible to state precisely how many children are born with intersex traits each year, some estimates run as high as 1 percent or more of all births. When children are born with genitalia that do not conform to the conventional male/female dichotomy, sometimes surgery is performed to make the genitals appear more like either those of a boy or of a girl, or to bring other organs (e.g., internal sex organs) closer to conformity with those expected in the binary model. By definition, an infant or very young child cannot consent to surgery, so the decision is typically made by the child's parents, in consultation with one or more physicians. The practice of surgically "correcting" nonconforming genitalia in infancy was popularized in part by Dr. John Money's reports of the case of David/Brenda Reimer in the 1960s. Although Reimer challenged Money's account of his life, and many consider Money's reports to be fraudulent, the practice of surgical "correction" on very young intersex children remains widespread, according to separate reports by the United Nations and by Human Rights Watch.

There is very little data available to guide this decision—for instance, no studies have been performed that make it possible to state if intersex children who have surgery as infants to make their genitals appear more conventionally male or female enjoy better or worse psychological adjustment in childhood and adulthood, if they have better or worse life outcomes, and so on. Given this lack of data, plus contemporary understanding about gender identity as independent of physical sex, means that many organizations and individuals now advocate delaying genital surgery unless strictly medically necessary (e.g., if the child cannot urinate properly) until the child has a clearly formed sense of gender and can make an informed choice to consent or decline the surgery.

"Corrective" surgery on intersex children may be irreversible, posing a problem if the gender assignment made in infancy does not match the individual's sense of gender identity as a child, adolescent, or adult. The United Nations condemns medically unnecessary surgery on intersex infants and children as a violation of the right to physical integrity and notes that such surgery may lead to many ill effects, including infertility, pain, loss of sexual sensation, and mental suffering. Human Rights Watch notes the lack of clear standards of care recognizing the rights of intersex children, and the legal and social limbo that may be faced by a child that is not assigned to one sex or the other. Human Rights Watch also notes that most parents want what is best for their child but may be unaware of the complexity of issues such as gender identity (as are many people for whom it has never been an issue). Parents may, therefore, rely on the advice of medical professionals who are similarly ill-informed and opt to "fix" their child without understanding all the potential consequences of that decision.

There are currently no studies comparing the outcomes for children who do or do not receive surgical or hormonal treatments at a young age, and hence no scientific evidence supporting early intervention. The closest analogue may be a study in Amsterdam that followed a group of transgender adolescents who received hormones to block the development of puberty at around age 13, cross-gender hormones at about age 16, and gender-reassignment surgery at about age 20. When evaluated in their early twenties, study participants were as mentally healthy as their cisgender peers. However, the participants in these studies were at least in early adolescence and were able to articulate their gender identity, quite a different situation from an infant who is neither able to express a sense of gender identity nor give consent to treatment.

HIV AND OTHER SEXUALLY TRANSMITTED DISEASES

United States

Transgender people are more likely than the general U.S. population to be living with HIV, according to data from the 2015 U.S. Transgender Survey. Overall, 1.4 percent of respondents were living with HIV, as compared to 0.3 percent in the general U.S. population. Transgender women were more likely to be living with HIV (3.4%) than were trans men (0.3%) or nonbinary individuals (0.4%). HIV status showed substantial variation at race and ethnicity, with blacks most likely to be living with HIV (6.7%), followed by American Indians (2.0%), Hispanics (1.6%), multiracial individuals (0.8%), and Asians (0.5%). HIV status varied by age, with those in the 45 to 64 years age group most likely to be living with HIV (3.3%), followed by those age 25 to 44 (2.0%), 65 and over (1.6%), and 18 to 24 (0.2%). Other variables associated with a high probability of living with HIV include being an undocumented resident (15.0%), working in the underground economy (15.0%), engaging in sex work at any time (7.9%), and not having completed high school (7.2%).

Respondents were much more likely to have been tested for HIV (55%) than the general U.S. adult population (34%). Transgender women were most likely to have been tested (62%), as compared to transgender men (58%) and nonbinary people (45%). Among racial and ethnic groups, blacks were most likely to have been tested (70%), followed by American Indians (65%), multiracial individuals (59%), Hispanics (54%), Middle Eastern individuals (53%), whites (52%), and Asians (49%). The rate of testing was substantially higher among those currently working in the underground economy (78%).

Most (87%) of the respondents living with HIV said they had received HIV-related care in the past month, and 89 percent said they had received HIV-related care from a doctor or healthcare provider in the last year. For those who had not received HIV-related care in the past six months or year, reasons stated included not having health insurance, not being able to afford care, not being ready to begin HIV care, not knowing where to go to receive care, not feeling sick enough to seek care, and relying on God or a higher power to deal with HIV.

Among those living with HIV, 82 percent had their blood tested in the past six months to determine their CD4 counts and viral load, 5 percent had received such testing between 6 and 12 months prior, 6 percent had been tested more than a year ago, and 7 percent had never been tested. A lower proportion (87%) reported being treated with antiretroviral therapy (ART), as compared to 94 percent of the total U.S. population living with HIV. Among those prescribed ART, 64 percent reported taking it as prescribed all the time, 33 percent taking it as prescribed most of the time, and 3 percent said they rarely or never took it as prescribed. Among those who were not always taking their ART medications as prescribed, the most common reason given (45%) was that they simply forgot to take it.

Tonia Poteat and colleagues reviewed the scientific literature concerning HIV infection and related conditions among transgender people, both in the United States and globally. They found 21 studies published between 2012 and 2015 that measured HIV prevalence (existing cases) among transgender people in the United States; one study also measured HIV incidence (new cases). The studies varied on many factors, including sample size (from 23 to 2,136), method of determining HIV status (self-report or laboratory confirmation), sampling method, age groups included, and population sample (some were national, some regional, some based in one or two cities), all factors that may help explain the differences found in the proportion of the sample infected with HIV.

Among trans female adults, Poteat and colleagues found prevalence ranging from 2.0 percent to 40.1 percent, and among trans female youths found HIV prevalence ranging from 4.5 percent to 7.9 percent. Among trans male individuals, the prevalence of HIV ranged from 0.9 percent to

4.3 percent. These differences underline the need for further research to understand the prevalence of HIV in different transgender communities and to be able to provide each with appropriate services.

There is no systematic surveillance of sexually transmitted diseases (STDs) among transgender people, although a number of research studies have examined this issue, usually with small, nonrandom samples. In 2012, the Substance Abuse and Mental Health Services Administration (SAMHSA) published a summary of research regarding STDs among transgender people in the United States. These studies find wide variance in the prevalence of STDs, at least some of which can be attributed to differences in sampling and other methodological concerns. In various studies, the rate of syphilis has been found to range from 3 to 79 percent, the rate of gonorrhea from 4 to 14 percent, the rate of chlamydia from 2 to 8 percent, the rate of herpes from 2 to 6 percent, and the rate of human papillomavirus (HPV) from 3 to 7 percent. Among transgender women, rates of hepatitis C ranging from 11 to 24 percent have been found by various studies, and rates of hepatitis from 4 to 76 percent.

Other Countries

There is little reliable data on transgender people and HIV outside North America. According to a 2015 policy brief from the World Health Organization (WHO), there are a variety of reasons for this lack of information, including problems in sampling, lack of information about the transgender population, and issues related to discrimination and stigma. Even if information is collected that indicates which respondents are transgender, often the number in that group is so small that it is aggregated with others groups when results are reported. Many national governments are also slowly recognizing transgender people as a group with distinct needs—for instance, only 39 percent of countries reported in 2014 that their national AIDS strategies address transgender people.

Most existing data concerns transgender women, because they tend to have a much higher burden of HIV than transgender men. As reported in the WHO policy brief, one systematic review and meta-analysis of data from 15 countries found that 19 percent of transgender women were HIV positive, 49 times higher than in the general population. A different meta-analysis found that transgender female sex workers had a 27 percent HIV infection rate, as compared to 15 percent among transgender women who were not sex workers. Neither study included data from countries in Eastern Europe or Africa, as no published data was available from either region at the time the research was conducted.

Many studies have found that transgender women suffer from high rates of many health and social problems that may make them particularly vulnerable to HIV infection, including violence, victimization, substance use, sexual abuse, and sexual assault. Depression, suicidal ideation, and suicide attempts have also been found to be high among transgender women, and they are often subject to structural and social inequalities including difficulties in obtaining appropriate identification documents, high rates of unemployment and underemployment, homelessness, lack of access to health care, and widespread discrimination and stigma. Those who engage in street sex work usually earn low pay and have little legal protection. Many have partners who are at high risk of HIV but may be willing to engage in sex without protection in return for psychological affirmation of their gender.

Fewer studies have reported on HIV prevalence among transgender men, and all have been conducted on populations from North America. A meta-analysis on this topic found only two studies in which HIV status was confirmed by lab tests: one found no HIV infections among the men, and the other found an infection rate of 2 percent. However, some studies have indicated that transgender men who have sex with men are at an increased risk for HIV infection.

Poteat and colleagues reviewed studies published between 2012 and 2015 that looked at HIV prevalence in transgender populations outside the United States. Only five studies examined HIV prevalence among trans male individuals; of these, two were conducted in Canada, one in Portugal, one in Spain, and one globally. The studies varied in sample size (from 14 to 227), method of sampling, and method of determining HIV status (laboratory test or self-report), which may account for some of the variation in HIV rates found. Prevalence of HIV infection in these five studies range from 2 percent to 8 percent.

Thirty-three studies reviewed by Poteat and colleagues looked at HIV prevalence among trans feminine individuals. These studies used a variety of methods of sampling and determination of HIV status, varied widely in sample size, and were conducted in many different countries (14 in Latin America and the Caribbean, 10 in Asia and the Pacific Islands, the remaining 9 in Europe, Canada, or multiple countries), all factors that may explain some of the variance in the rates of HIV infection found. The rate of HIV infection found in individual studies ranged from 0 percent to 45.2 percent.

CHAPTER 5

Mental Health

Trans people face a variety of mental health issues, some of which are similar to those faced by cisgender people and others that are specific to their trans status, and others that may be exacerbated by the discrimination and social disapproval they face. For instance, suicidal ideation, suicide attempts, and suicide are higher among trans people than in the general population, and like many other mental health issues, social disadvantage is generally associated with increased risk of suicide. Given the discrimination and social exclusion faced by many trans people on a daily basis, it is not surprising that a high proportion of the trans population are dealing with mental health issues, as compared to the U.S. population as a whole, not that many have unmet mental health needs.

OVERALL MENTAL HEALTH

United States

Based on the evidence presented by the 2015 National Transgender Survey, the lives of transgender individuals in the United States are more likely to be impacted by psychological distress than are the lives of individuals in the U.S. population as a whole. Psychological distress in the Transgender Survey was measured using the Kessler Psychological Distress Scale, also known as the K6, which asked respondents to rate how often they have experienced feelings of psychological distress, such as hopelessness or worthlessness, over the past month. Respondents are also asked to indicate how often they have experienced each feeling, on a five-point scale ranging from "none of the time" to "all of the time." Looking

at those who indicated that they had felt at least one of the feelings of psychological distress (i.e., everyone who did not select "none of the time"
for all the feelings of distress), 29 percent of the transgender respondents
indicated "a lot" of interference with their life and activities due to psychological distress in the past 30 days, 35 indicated "some" interference,
26 percent "a little" interference, and 10 percent said their feelings of
psychological distress interfered "not at all" with their life and activities.
These levels of reported inference with life and activities are much higher
than reported for the general U.S. population as measured by the National
Health Interview Survey (NHIS), in which 12 percent reported "a lot" of
interference, 22 percent "some" interference, 31 percent "a little" interference, and 35 percent said psychological distress affected their life and
activities "not at all."

A variable developed from the K6 to indicate if an individual was experiencing current serious psychological distress also indicated that individuals in the transgender sample were more bothered by psychological
distress than the NHIS sample of the general U.S. population. Among
respondents to the National Transgender Survey, 39 percent reported
experiencing serious psychological distress, as compared to 5 percent
of the general population. Within the transgender sample, cross-dressers
reported the least serious psychological distress (18%), while 35 percent
of transgender men and women indicated serious psychological distress,
as did 49 percent of nonbinary individuals. Younger individuals within
the transgender sample were more likely than older individuals to experience serious psychological distress, with the highest level reported in the
18–25-year-old group (53%).

As in the general population, levels of distress generally declined
with age, although within every age group, higher levels of distress were
reported within the transgender sample as compared to the general population. For those age 26 to 29, 39 percent reported serious psychological
distress, as did 31 percent of those age 30 to 34, 26 percent of those age
35 to 39, 23 percent of those age 40 to 44, 22 percent of those age 45 to
49, 16 percent of those age 50 to 54, 14 percent of those age 55 to 59,
10 percent of those age 60 to 64, and 8 percent of those age 65 and older.
Low levels of education were also associated with higher probability of
currently experiencing serious psychological distress. Among those who
did not complete high school, 58 percent reported serious psychological
distress; among high school graduates, 54 percent; for those with some
college, 48 percent; for those with an associate's degree, 32 percent, for
those with a bachelor's degree, 30 percent; and for those with a graduate
or professional degree, 18 percent. Levels of distress were higher among

those who wanted to transition but had not done so (49%) or had transitioned within the past year (41%), as compared to those who transitioned 2 to 5 years ago (38%), 6 to 10 years ago (31%), and 10 years or more previously (24%). Levels of distress were also higher than average for people living in poverty (52%), living with a disability (59%), who had been fired or denied a promotion in the past year due to their status (51%), and who had been physically (59%) or sexually assaulted (60%) in the past year.

Canada

Most respondents to the Canadian Trans Youth Health Survey, conducted among young people age 14–25, reported relatively low levels of mental health: only 3 percent indicated their mental health was excellent, 31 percent good, 45 percent fair, and 22 percent poor. Younger respondents (age 14–28) were also asked how often they had felt happy in the previous 30 days: only 2 percent said they had felt happy all of the time, 22 percent most of the time, 41 percent some of the time, 29 percent a little of the time, and 6 percent none of the time.

Many trans youth also reported high levels of stress on this survey. Among younger youth, asked about the level of stress they had felt in the past 30 days, 44 percent saying they felt so stressed they could not do their work or deal with things, 29 percent said they felt quite a bit of stress, 17 percent said they felt some stress, 8 percent a little stress, and 2 percent said they were not stressed at all. Older youth were asked a slightly different question, in which they were asked to characterize most days of their life. Nine percent said most days were extremely stressful, 39 percent quite a bit stressful, 43 percent a bit stressful, as compared to only 8 percent who felt their days were not very stressful and 2 percent who felt their days were not at all stressful.

UNMET NEEDS

Many respondents to the 2015 National Transgender Survey reported unmet needs in their transition-related health care. For instance, 77 percent said they wanted counseling or therapy related to their gender identity or gender transition, but only 58 percent had received such therapy. The desire for such counseling was only somewhat higher among transgender men and women (81%) than among nonbinary individuals (70%), but transgender men and women were much more likely to have received such counseling (73%) as compared to nonbinary individuals (31%). Higher income was strongly related to success in receiving counseling and therapy, with only 39 percent of those reporting no income having received counseling and therapy, 48 percent of those with incomes from $1 to $999, 59 percent of those with incomes from $10,000 to $24,999, 70 percent of those with incomes from $24,000 to $49,999, and 76 percent of those with incomes of $50,000 or more.

Among the younger (age 14–18) trans youth who took part in the Canadian Trans Youth Health Survey, two-thirds (68%) reported not accessing mental health care at least once when they needed it in the past year (the question was not asked of old trans youths). Among the most common reasons given for not accessing needed mental health care were not wanting parents to know (71%), thinking or hoping the problem would go away (62%), being afraid of what the doctor would say or do (54%), having had negative experiences before (43%), and not knowing where to go (43%).

GENDER DYSPHORIA/GENDER IDENTITY DISORDER

The terms *gender dysphoria* and *gender identity disorder* are both used to refer to a condition in which an individual's gender identity does not correspond with their gender as assigned at birth. The fifth edition of the *Diagnostic and Statistical Manual of Mental Disorders* (*DSM-5*) uses the term *gender dysphoria*, while the fourth edition used the term *identity disorder*, and both terms remain in use in current medical and psychiatric practice. Persons with gender dysphoria may feel uncomfortable with their assigned gender or their body and may experience significant distress as a result. However, gender dysphoria is not the same as gender nonconformity, which refers to individuals behaving or dressing in ways culturally associated with the opposite sex (e.g., girls may want to wear boys' clothing or participate in sports such as American football that are usually played by males). Gender dysphoria is also not the same as being gay or lesbian, which is a matter of sexual preference rather than gender identity.

Individuals with gender dysphoria may react in different ways. Some may want to present an appearance consonant with their gender identity—for instance, by wearing clothing and hairstyles considered appropriate to the gender with which they identify. Some may want to socially transition, which can include changes such as asking others to use pronouns appropriate to their gender identity and using facilities such as public restrooms appropriate to that identity. Some may want to medically transition, using hormone treatments, surgery, or other methods to change their body.

In the *DSM-5*, the criteria for diagnosis of gender dysphoria in children requires that the individual experience "a marked incongruence between one's experienced/expressed gender and assigned gender" lasting at least six months, and that the individual have at least six of eight symptoms from a list. Examples of the qualifying symptoms, many of which are based on observable behavior, are insisting one is of the other gender (or some alternative gender) from that assigned at birth, strongly preferring to dress in clothing associated with the opposite sex, and strongly disliking one's sexual anatomy. *DSM-5* also notes that gender dysphoria is typically associated with significant distress or impairment in important areas of functioning, such as school.

For adolescents and adults, diagnosis of gender dysphoria also requires that the individual experience a strong incongruence between their assigned and felt gender for at least six months, but the list of symptoms is different, focusing less on observable behaviors and more on felt incongruence between somatic sex and felt gender. To be diagnosed with gender dysphoria, adolescents and adults need to display only two of the six symptoms, which include a desire to get rid of primary or secondary sexual characteristics, or to prevent their expression in the case of young adolescents; a desire for the sex characteristics of the opposite gender; and a conviction that one has feelings and reactions typical of the opposite or some alternative gender rather than one's assigned gender.

DSM-5 lists several conditions that should be differentiated from gender dysphoria. Simple nonconformity to gender roles includes cases such as a girl acting like a tomboy or an adult man occasionally wearing women's clothing. *Transvestic disorder* refers to individuals (usually heterosexual or bisexual adolescent or adult males) who achieve sexual excitement through cross-dressing. Body dysmorphic disorder means that an individual believes a specific body part is malformed and should be removed, but not because it is experienced as incongruous for their gender. Individuals with schizophrenic or other psychotic disorders may have a delusion of belonging to another gender, but believing one is of the opposite sex is not by itself sufficient to make a diagnosis of schizophrenia.

Several comorbidities are more common in children with a diagnosis of gender dysphoria than in those without it, including anxiety, depressive, and disruptive and impulse-control disorders. Before the onset of puberty, increased age is associated with increased behavioral and emotional problems, possibly due to increasing ostracism by peers who perceive the individual to be displaying non-gender-appropriate behavior. Autism spectrum disorder is more common among children and adolescents diagnosed with gender dysphoria. Common comorbidities among adults with gender dysphoria include depressive disorders and anxiety.

Not all children who identify as transgender when they are young keep that status as they grow up. James Cantor summarized 11 studies, books, and dissertations published between 1972 and 2013 that tracked a number of children who were identified as transgender when they were young and followed them into adulthood. The studies vary in terms of the size of the population, the terminology and definitions used, the age of the children studied, the types of outcomes collected (e.g., some indicate which transgender children became gay adults, while others only indicate transgender or cisgender status in adulthood), and in other ways, making it difficult to combine data from them. However, it is clear that most of the transgender children studied did not become transgender adults.

The two largest studies used samples of 139 and 127 individuals. In the study with the larger sample, 12.2 percent became transgender adults, the remaining cisgender adults. In the study with the smaller sample, 37.0 percent became transgender adults, the remainder cisgender adults. In the remaining studies, with sample sizes from 8 to 54, in one none of the children became transgender adults, while in another, 38.9 percent did. The percentage of children who became gay, lesbian, or bisexual adults (among the studies which recorded that information) ranged from 100 percent to 4.5 percent. Given the variability in outcomes, the safest conclusion to draw is that a transgender child may or may not grow up to be a transgender adult, and the probability of either outcome is unknown.

CONVERSION THERAPY

Conversion therapy attempts to change someone's gender or sexual orientation or identity—for instance, to make a homosexual person into a heterosexual person, or to convince a transgender person that they are in fact the gender they were assigned at birth. Some advocates of conversion therapy base their arguments on a religion, usually Christianity, and/or on psychoanalytic theories no longer embraced by the majority of the medical or psychological community, but neither form of justification is required in conversion therapy. Proponents of conversion therapy typically reject the scientific consensus that human sexuality and gender expression can be varied, instead considering any deviations from what they consider to be the norm to be defects or bad behavior rather than a fundamental aspect of an individual's identity.

Jack Drescher and colleagues summarize the many ethical objections made to conversion therapy in practice. These include telling a patient that homosexuality is a disorder, based on the provider opinion rather than referring to the consensus view of the medical and psychological community that it is not; breaching patient confidentiality, for example, informing others of a patient's homosexuality; placing improper pressure on patients to submit to the therapist's authority; refusing to refer patients to a gay-affirmative therapy after conversion therapy fails; persisting in offering a treatment without regard for the probability of success; and blaming the patient for failure to change their sexuality. Being subjected to conversion therapy can have negative psychological outcomes for the patient, including anxiety, depression, suicidal ideation, and acquisition of negative stereotypes about homosexuality. In addition, if a patient is encouraged to marry a member of the opposite sex and have a family, despite being homosexual, then the spouse and children may be harmed by this deception.

As of January 2017, conversion therapy has been outlawed in four U.S. states (California, New Jersey, Oregon, and Illinois) and two Canadian provinces (Manitoba and Ontario), although in some cases the ban only applies to minor patients. Despite this, and the consensus view of the medical and psychological communities that conversion therapy is both ineffective and harmful, it is still offered by some counselors, psychologists, and psychiatrists, and some transgender people still seek it out. Even if transgender persons are secure in their transgender identity, they may feel the need to suppress it in order to delay their transition in order to avoid rejection by family members, discrimination in employment or others facets of life, or to bring themselves more in line with the proclamations of their religion.

Among respondents to the 2015 National Transgender Survey, 13 percent reported attempts by at least one professional (e.g., a psychologist or religious adviser) to stop them from being transgender. This experience was most common among Middle Eastern individuals (32%) and American Indians (27%), and less common among multiracial individuals (21%), whites (19%), Hispanics (17%), blacks (16%), and Asians (14%). Among individuals who had experienced a professional trying to stop them from being transgender, 47 percent experienced serious psychological distress, 58 percent had attempted suicide, 22 percent had run away from home, 46 percent had been homeless at some point in their life, and 18 percent had done sex work at some point in their life; in every case, the proportion of these negative factors was higher for those who had had this experience than for those who had not.

SUICIDE

United States

Many studies have found that rates of suicidal ideation, suicide attempts, and suicide are higher among transgender people than in the general population. These statistics should not be interpreted as signs that transgender people are inherently unstable; however, it is also possible that suicide is a response to the lived experience of discrimination and abuse, and a reflection of inadequate medical and psychiatric care. Almost half (48%) of respondents to the 2015 U.S. National Transgender Survey indicated that they had seriously thought of killing themselves in the past 12 months, and 7 percent had attempted suicide in the past year; by comparison, the comparable figures for the general U.S. population are 7 percent (suicidal thoughts) and 1.1 percent (attempted suicide). The rate of suicide among transgender responders was higher among people with disabilities (12%), American Indians (10%), multiracial individuals (10%), blacks (9%), and Hispanics (9%).

Lower levels of education are associated with increased risk for attempting suicide among respondents to the National Transgender Survey. Among those who did not complete high school, 17 attempted suicide in the past year, as compared to 13 percent for high school graduates, 9 percent for people with some college education, 6 percent for people with an associate's degree, 4 percent for those with a bachelor's degree, and 3 percent for those with a graduate or professional degree. Attempted suicide was more common in younger age groups: among those aged 18–25, 10 percent attempted suicide in the past year, as compared to 7 percent of those aged 20–29, 5 percent of those aged 30–34 and 25–39, 4 percent of those aged 40–44, 3 percent of those aged 45–49 and 50–54, 2 percent of those aged 55–59 and 60–64, and 1 percent of those aged 65 and over.

Canada

Respondents to the Canadian Trans Youth Health Survey reported high levels of discouragement and hopelessness, both of which can be risk factors for suicide. Younger trans people (aged 14–18) were asked if they "felt so discouraged, hopeless, or have so many problems they wonder if anything was worthwhile in the past month." Twenty-eight percent said that they felt "extremely so, to the point where I couldn't do my work or deal with things," while another 21 percent said they felt that way "quite a bit." Among older trans youth (aged 19–25), almost three-quarters (71%) said they had felt "sad, blue, or depressed" for at least two consecutive weeks. More than half of both age groups felt they had deliberately hurt themselves in the past month without wanting to die (self-harm), although was more common among the younger age group (75%) than the older (51%).

In the younger age group, 65 percent said they had seriously considered suicide in the past 12 months, and 37 percent had made at least one suicide attempt during that time; 19 percent had attempted suicide once, 12 percent two or three times, 5 percent four or five times, and 2 percent six or more times. In the older age group, 69 percent reported having seriously considered suicide at least once in their life, and 37 percent said they had attempted suicide at least once.

A 2011 survey conducted by TRANS Pulse of 433 individuals aged 16 or older who live, work, or receive health care in Ontario found that 10 percent of respondents had attempted suicide within the past year, and 43 had attempted suicide within their lifetime. The percentage that had attempted suicide within the past year was much higher for those who had been the victims of a physical or sexual assault (29%), as compared to only 4 percent among those who had not experienced any type of harassment (physical, sexual, or verbal). Overall, 35 percent of respondents had considered seriously suicide in the past year, but for those who had experienced physical or sexual assault, 56 percent had considered suicide in the past year. Among respondents aged 16–24 with supportive parents, only 4 percent attempted suicide in the previous year, as compared to 57 percent of those without good parental support.

Research reported by Greta R. Bauer and colleagues, based on the Trans PULSE survey conducted in Ontario, many factors associated with higher risk of suicide among transgender people are modifiable through policy, social, or medical interventions. These factors fell into three main groups: social inclusion, transphobia (including internalized stigma), and sex or gender transition. Factors included in the social inclusion category are increased social support, strong support for gender identity and expression, increased religiosity or spirituality, and identity document concordance. Factors included within transphobia are reduced transphobic experiences and reduced transphobic violence. Factors included within sex or gender transition are medical transition, hormone treatment, social transition, and being socially read as cisgender.

Bauer and colleagues calculate the expected reduction in suicidal ideation and suicide attempts within the Trans PULSE sample, if changes were made in the intervenable factors. Some of these changes were quite impressive—for instance, a high level of social support, as compared to a low level, was associated with a 49 percent reduction in suicidal ideation and an 82 percent reduction in suicide attempts among those with considering suicide. This research suggests that suicidal ideation and suicide attempts among transgender youth could be sharply reduced if resources were made available to make changes in these modifiable factors.

ALCOHOL, TOBACCO, AND SUBSTANCE ABUSE

United States

Only limited studies have been conducted regarding the use of alcohol, tobacco, and illegal drugs among transgender people, and the small, non-random samples used in some studies means that it is difficult to draw any conclusions from them regarding the transgender population as a whole. A report from the Substance Abuse and Mental Health Services Administration found that some studies have found rates of tobacco use as high as 74 percent among transgender people. High rates of other substances of abuse have also been found in some transgender populations; for instances, rates of methamphetamine use as high as 46 percent in some samples, and injection drug use rates as high as 40 percent. Some studies, as reported by the Program for LGBTI Health of the Vanderbilt University School of Medicine, have found elevated rates of alcohol use and abuse among transgender people as well.

Judging by the results of the 2015 U.S. Transgender National Transgender Survey, transgender people are more likely to use a number of substances, including alcohol, tobacco, and various drugs of abuse, as compared to the general U.S. population. This information should not be used to judge the transgender community, however, but should be interpreted in light of the knowledge that transgender people face many stresses that the average person does not, and often have greater difficulty finding appropriate medical care, so that substance use may be one way to try to cope with those stresses or to self-medicate in the absence of adequate medical care.

Alcohol use as reported by respondents to the National Transgender Survey was only slightly higher than that of the general U.S. adult population. Almost all respondents (90%) reported having drunk alcohol at some point in their lives, as compared to 86 percent of the general U.S. adult population who say they have consumed alcohol at least once. Sixty-three percent of respondents said they were current drinkers, defined as having consumed at least one alcoholic beverage in the last 30 days, also slightly higher than the proportion of the general U.S. adult population reporting this behavior (56%). The rate of binge drinking, defined as consuming five or more alcoholic drinks on the same occasion within the past month, was also slightly higher (27%) than in the general U.S. adult population (25%).

A lower percentage of respondents to the survey (57%) reported having ever smoked in their lives, as compared to the general U.S. adult population (63%). Twenty-two percent of respondents were current smokers, meaning they had smoked within the past 30 days, as compared to 21 percent of the general population. However, current smoking was much more common among survey respondents working in the underground economy (e.g., sex work, selling drugs): among those individuals, 51 percent were current tobacco users.

Marijuana use was substantially higher among survey respondents than in the general U.S. adult population: 64 percent of survey respondents reported having ever used marijuana, as compared to 47 percent in the general population. Twenty-five percent of respondents reported current marijuana use (having smoked in the past 30 days), as compared to 8 percent of the general population, and marijuana use was higher among respondents with HIV (48%) or who worked in the underground economy (60%).

Twenty-nine percent of survey respondents reported having used illegal or illicit drugs (e.g., cocaine, crack, LSD, or inhalants, but not including marijuana) in their lifetimes, and 4 percent reported having used such drugs at least once in the past 30 days (current use). Lifetime use of illicit or illegal drugs was higher among those who had done sex work (56%), worked in the underground economy (75%), had lost a job because they were transgender (43%), or had even been homeless (42%). Current illicit drug use was almost nine times as high (26%) among those currently working in the underground economy, as compared to those not currently working in the underground economy (3%).

About one-third (34%) of survey respondents report nonmedical use of prescription drugs (OxyContin, Adderall, Xanax, etc.) at some point in their lifetime. Nonmedical prescription drug use was much higher among those who worked in the underground economy (63%) and was most common in the 25 to 44 age group (39%). Over half (51%) reporting lifetime nonmedical use of prescription drugs reported using them in the past year, and 21 percent reported using them in the past 30 days. This corresponds to 7 percent of all survey respondents reporting nonmedical use of prescription drugs in the past 30 days, a much higher percentage than for the U.S. population as a whole (2%).

Canada

Many respondents to the Canadian Trans Youth Health Survey report having used tobacco, alcohol, or other legal or illegal drugs. Among older youths (aged 19–25), almost half (49%) reporting that they had smoked at least one whole cigarette. Of those who have ever smoked, 20 percent were currently daily smokers, 32 percent smoke occasionally, and 48 percent did not currently smoke at all. Only a third of young youths reported ever using tobacco; among those who had, 26 percent report smoking cigarettes in the past 30 days, 10 percent each smoking cigars, cigarillos, or electronic cigarettes with nicotine, 4 percent smoking a hookah, and 1 percent using chewing tobacco (respondents could indicate more than one category of tobacco use).

Just under half of those in the younger age group reporting drinking alcohol in the previous 12 months, with 20 percent reporting binge drinking (five or more drinks on one occasion) at least once in the previous month. Over three-quarters of older youths said they had consumed alcohol at least once in the past year, with 27 percent drinking at least once a week, and 53 percent binge drinking at least once in the past year. Among older trans youth who drank, 7 percent said they first drank alcohol when they were 11 years old or young, 31 percent when they were aged 12–14, 43 percent when they were aged 15–17, and 19 percent when they were aged 18 or older.

Almost half (46%) of the younger age group said they had used marijuana at least once, and more than one-third (36%) reported having used it in the previous 12 months. In the older age group, over two-thirds (69%) had used marijuana at least once, and 8 percent had used it on a daily basis over the past year. Sixteen percent of the total sample reported using marijuana on the previous Saturday night (12% of the younger age group, 18% of the older age group).

Trans youth also reported using a variety of other drugs and substances of abuse. Among the younger age group, 17 percent reporting using prescription drugs not prescribed for them (e.g., Ritalin, OxyContin) at least once in the past 12 months, 14 percent reported using Ecstasy (MDMA), 12 percent inhalants (e.g., glue, nitrous oxide), 11 percent hallucinogens, 10 percent mushrooms, and 7 percent cocaine. In the older age group, 14 percent reported using Ecstasy at least once in the past 12 months, 13 percent hallucinogens, 8 percent cocaine, 6 percent amphetamines, 1 percent solvents (e.g., glue, gasoline), and 1 percent heroin.

PART II

Controversies and Issues

CHAPTER 6

Discrimination against Transgender People

Many transgender people face discrimination, harassment, and mistreatment on a regular basis, in venues ranging from schools to places of employment to the criminal justice system. These experiences can range from verbal harassment to physical attack, and in some cases discrimination inbuilt into the law—for instance, trans people were barred from military service in the United States until 2016, although many in fact served before that time. Trans people also face issues with credentialing—that is, obtaining legal forms of identification (such as a driver's license) that accurately reflects their gender identity.

GENERAL EXPERIENCES OF HARASSMENT

United States

According to the 2015 U.S. Transgender Survey, conducted by the National Center for Transgender Equality, transgender people often experience harassment, discrimination, and mistreatment, factors that have been shown to be negatively related to many aspects of well-being, including health. Over half (54%) of respondents reported being verbally harassed in the past year and most (85%) of those reporting harassment attributed it to their transgender status, so 46 percent of respondents reported harassment based on their transgender status. The experience of verbal harassment was highest (70%) among those working in the underground economy, and among those identifying as Middle Eastern (67%), multiracial (66%), or American Indian (65%).

Discrimination was less commonly reported, with 16 percent reporting they had been denied equal treatment or service in the past year; 14 percent, or 88 percent of those reporting discrimination, said the denial was due to their transgender status. Denial of equal treatment was more common (24%) among those who said that others could always or usually tell that they were transgender, as compared to 10 percent among those who said others could rarely or never tell that they were transgender. Denial of equal treatment was also higher among those working in the underground economy (33%), and among persons of color, including those identifying as American Indian (30%), Middle Eastern (23%), multiracial (2%), and black (20%).

The National Transgender Discrimination Survey also found a high level of harassment and discrimination against transgender individuals. Over half (53%) of respondents reported being verbally harassed or disrespected in public, with the highest levels of harassment reported among those who were visually nonconforming (64%), were living full-time in their trans identity (59%), identified as female-to-male (62%), were working in the underground economy (77%), or identified as multiracial (65%). Just under half (44%) of respondents reported discrimination or lack of equal treatment in at least one public accommodation, with higher rates reported among those identifying as female-to-male (50%), with income of $20,000 or less (53%), who were visually nonconforming (53%), and who identified as multiracial (57%), Hispanic (50%), or American Indian (49%).

Europe

Many transgender people in Europe experience discrimination or harassment, according to the results of the 2014 European Union Lesbian, Gay, Bisexual and Transgender Survey, with almost half (46%) reporting they had personally experienced harassment or discrimination in the past year, based on their status. In addition, 84 percent said that they felt that discrimination against sexual minorities because of their status was "fairly or very widespread," a higher percentage than for the other sexual minorities included in the sample (by way of comparison, 36 percent of bisexual men or women, 52 percent of lesbians, and 73 percent of gay men felt such discrimination was "fairly or very widespread").

EDUCATION

United States

Many transgender students in grades 6–12 in the United States experience the school climate as threatening, according to the 2015 National School Climate Survey. The study was conducted with students who self-identify as a sexual minority (lesbian, gay, bisexual, transgender, queer), and while most of the study is not broken down by the sexual identity of the student, many report hearing negative remarks about transgender people while in school. For instance, 85.7 percent of student report hearing negative remarks like "tranny" or "he/she" about transgender people, with 40.5 percent reporting hearing them often. Among transgender respondents, 50.9 percent said they were prevented from using their preferred name or pronoun, and 60.0 percent reported being required to use a bathroom or locker room that reflected the sex on their birth certificate rather than their gender identity.

Various reforms and programs were associated with lower rates of harassment. For instance, students attending a school with a Gay-Straight Alliance (GSA) or similar club reported hearing such remarks less often: in all schools, 46.0 percent of students report hearing negative remarks about transgender people often or frequently, as compared to 35.9 percent in schools with a GSA. Students attending a school with an LGBTQ-inclusive curriculum were less likely (26.8%) to report hearing negative remarks about transgender people, as compared to students in schools without such a curriculum (44.5%). Of course, the presence of a GSA or LGBTQ-inclusive curriculum may be a product of a deliberate attempt to reduce harassment, rather than a cause of it, but it is worth noting that harassment is not equally common in all schools.

According to the 2015 U.S. Transgender Survey, negative experiences in school are common among transgender individuals and those perceived as transgender. Among those who said they revealed their transgender status or were perceived by classmates, teachers, or school staff as gay, 77 percent said they had at least one negative experience in school in grades K-12 (kindergarten, elementary school, and high school). Experience of harassment was even higher among people with disabilities (82%) and among those who were American Indian (92%), Middle Eastern (84%), or multiracial (81%).

Negative experiences reported by those who revealed their transgender status or were perceived as transgender include being verbally harassed (54%), not being allowed to dress in a way that matched their gender identity or expression (52%), being disciplined for fighting back against bullies (36%), being physically attacked (24%), being disciplined by teachers or staff due to the discipliner's belief that they were transgender (20%), and being sexually assaulted because they were believed to be transgender (6%). Seventeen percent report they left school due to mistreatment and 6 percent said they were expelled from school. The experience of physical attack was most common among trans women (38%), as compared to cross-dressers (26%), trans men (20%), and nonbinary individuals, and trans women were also most likely to report sexual assault (21%), as compared to cross-dressers (18%), nonbinary individuals (10%), and trans men (9%). Trans women were also more likely to have left school due to mistreatment (22%) and to have been expelled from school (10%) than the average of all transgender individuals.

Levels of harassment were lower in higher education institutions, although still disturbingly high. Among respondents who attended college or vocational school, 24 percent reported being verbally, physically, or sexually harassed, and 16 percent reported leaving school due to harassment. The experience of harassment was highest among American Indians (37%), followed by blacks (28%), Middle Eastern individuals (27%), multiracial individuals (25%), white and Hispanics (each 23%), and Asians (22%). There was also substantial variation by race and ethnicity among those who left school due to harassment: American Indians and Hispanics (each 23%) were most likely to report doing this, followed by blacks (21%) and multiracial individuals (20%), while white (13%) and Asian (9%) individuals were much less likely to report leaving school due to harassment.

Canada

Among the respondents to the Canadian Trans Youth Health Survey, the average respondent felt little connection to his or her school: on a scale of 0 to 10, based on answers to questions such as "I am happy to be at my school" and "I feel close to people at my school," respondents scored an average of 4.9, with average scores noticeably higher in British Columbia (5.6) and Quebec (6.0), and lower in the "Atlantic Provinces" of New Brunswick, Prince Edward Island, Nova Scotia, and Newfoundland and Labrador (3.7) and the "Prairie Provinces" of Alberta, Saskatchewan, and Manitoba (4.1).

Despite this low sense of connectedness with school, most younger (aged 14–18) trans youth said they plan to continue in school, and over half anticipated post-high school education as well. In this age group, only 7 percent were not currently in school, and another 4 percent said they would like to quit school as soon as they can. In contrast, 20 percent planned to finish high school, 6 percent planned to attend vocational or trade school after high school, 52 percent wanted to attend college or university, and 11 percent said they would like to attend graduate or professional school after college or university. Older youth (aged 19–25) were also likely to be involved in education, with 45 percent indicating that their main activity in the past 12 months had been going to school, as compared to 32 percent who said it was working at a paid job or business.

Most trans students felt safe at school, with an average score of 6.5 on a scale where 0 means never feeling safe and 10 means always feeling safe. Students felt most safe in the library (42 percent always feel safe there) and in classrooms (29 percent always feel safe there), and least safe in locker rooms (only 5 percent always feel safe there, while 44 percent rarely or never feel safe there) and restrooms (only 10 percent always feel safe there, while 40 percent rarely or never feel safe there). Still, over half (55%) in the younger age group said they had been bullied at least once in school, while 24 percent said they had been bullied 1 to 3 times in the past year, and 13 percent had been bullied 12 or more times in the past year. Thirty-six percent of young participants said they had been physically threatened or injured in the past year, and 9 percent had been threatened or injured with a weapon.

Europe

Twenty percent of transgender respondents to the 2014 European Union Lesbian, Gay, Bisexual and Transgender Survey reported experiencing discrimination by school or university personnel in the past year. However, all respondents to the survey were at least 18 years old, so few would have been enrolled in education below the tertiary level in the past year. As a measure of discrimination in primary and secondary education, it is notable that 70 percent said they "always" or "often" hid or disguised their status while in school before the age of 18, suggesting they felt the need to conceal their identity to avoid harassment. Twenty-seven percent said they were "often" the recipient of negative comments or conducts at school because of their status, and 11 percent said they were "always" recipients of such comments or conduct.

EMPLOYMENT

United States

Transgender people often suffer from discrimination in the work place and are also more likely to be unemployed or to live in poverty than the U.S. population as a whole. According to the 2015 U.S. National Transgender Survey, among individuals who had even been employed (81 percent of the sample), 16 percent reported losing a job based on their gender identity or gender expression. This experience was more common among American Indians (21%), multiracial individuals (18%), blacks (17%), and Middle Eastern individuals (14%), and was less common among whites (12%), Hispanics (11%), and Asians (8%). Losing a job based on one's transgender status was most common among trans women (18%), followed by trans men (14%), nonbinary individuals (7%), and cross-dressers (3%).

Employment discrimination can take many forms, and overall 67 percent of respondents who had applied for a job in the past year reported experiencing some kind of discrimination based on their status. Among those who were not hired for a job they had applied for, 39 percent said they believed the reason was their gender identity or expression. Among those who had been denied a promotion in the past year, almost half (49%) said they believed it was due to their gender identity or expression, and among those fired in the past year, 43 percent said they believed the reason was their gender identity or expression. Among those who believed they were fired due to their gender identity or expression, 69 percent did nothing, 15 percent contacted a lawyer, 14 percent made an official complaint, 10 percent contacted a transgender, LGBT, or other group, 2 percent contacted their union representative, and 7 percent took some other action.

Among transgender people who had been employed in the past year, almost one-quarter (23 percent) reported experiencing mistreatment at work due to their transgender status. The most common complaint was that someone at work shared information about them that the individual should have kept confidential (16%; other complaints based on an individual's transgender status included a negative job review (6%), being forced to resign (4%), not being allowed to use the restroom corresponding to their gender identity (4%), being told they must present in their birth gender to keep their job (4%), being removed from direct contact with clients, customers, or patients (3%), being unable to work out an acceptable restroom situation (3%), and being forced to transfer to a different position or department (2%).

Over three-quarters (77%) reported taking some action to avoid transgender discrimination at work in the past year. The most common actions were to hide their gender identity (53%) or to not request the use of preferred pronouns (27%). Other responses included delaying gender transition (26%), staying in a job they would prefer to leave (26%), hiding a completed gender transition (25%), remaining in a job for which they were overqualified (24%), quitting a job (15%), not seeking a promotion or raise (13%), and requesting a transfer (6%). People living in poverty (82%) were most likely to report taking one of these actions, as were people with disabilities and nonbinary individuals (each 81%).

Unemployment among transgender people is three times as high (15%) as among the general population (5%), and transgender people are also over twice as likely to live in poverty (29%), as compared to the general U.S. population (29%). The highest rates of poverty among transgender individuals were reported by Hispanics (43%), American Indians (41%), and multiracial individuals (40%), followed by blacks (38%), Middle Eastern individuals (34%), Asians (32%), and whites (24%).

As compared to the general U.S. population, transgender people were overrepresented in lower income brackets and underrepresented in higher income brackets. Four percent of respondents to the transgender survey reported no household income, as compared to 1 percent in the general population; 12 percent of transgender people and 4 percent of the general population reported household income of $1 to $9,999; 22 percent of transgender individuals and 12 percent of the general population reported household income between $10,000 and $24,999; 24 percent of transgender individuals and 21 percent of the general population reported household income between $25,000 and $49,999; 23 percent of transgender individuals and 31 percent of the general population reported household income between $50,000 and $99,999; and only 15 percent of transgender individuals reported household income of $100,000 or more, as compared to 31 percent of the general population.

Canada

A 2015 report by Jaimie Veale and colleagues, based on a national online survey with 923 participants from all 10 Canadian provinces and 1 territory, summarized the experiences of individuals aged 14–25 who identified as transgender. Among respondents, 13 percent said they had been fired from a job due to their transgender status, and another 15 percent suspected that their transgender status was the cause of their being fired. Eighteen percent reported being turned for a job due to the transgender status, 17 percent turned down a job they had been offered because they felt it did not offer a safe environment for a transgender person, and another 32 percent suspected they had been turned down for a job based on their transgender status.

Europe

Discrimination in employment on the basis of sexual orientation is prohibited in European Union by several directives, including the Employment Equality Directive of 2000 and the Gender Equality Directive. However, discrimination remains a common experience for sexual minorities, with 30 percent of transgender respondents to the 2014 European Union Lesbian, Gay, Bisexual and Transgender Survey said they had been discriminated in the past year while looking for a job, and 23 percent reporting discrimination while on the job. These levels of discrimination are even higher than the average for the entire survey sample, which included lesbian, gay, and bisexual people as well; for the total sample, 13 percent said they had been discriminated against in the past year while looking for work, and 19 percent while on the job. Transgender people were also more likely to report negative comments, attitudes, or unequal treatment at work, with 15 percent saying they had this experience often, and 4 percent always; for the total sample, only 8 percent said they had such experiences often, and 1 percent always.

Perhaps because of higher levels of discrimination and negative experiences, transgender people were less likely than the total sample to be open about their status at work. Among transgender respondents, 49 percent said they had never been open about their status at work, as compared to 23 percent of the total sample; 21 percent of transgender respondents said they were rarely open at work, as compared to 23 percent of the total sample; 13 percent of transgender recipients said they were often open at work, compared to 20 percent of the total sample, and 17 percent said they were always open at work, compared to 23 percent of the total sample.

MILITARY SERVICE

Prior to June 30, 2016, transgender people were openly barred from serving in the U.S. military. Despite this, research has found that transgender people serve in the military at a higher rate than the general U.S. population. Data from the 2015 U.S. National Transgender Survey, collected while transgender people were barred from serving openly, confirms this finding, and also indicates that the status of some transgender people was known while they were serving in the military, despite the prohibitions then in place. Overall, 15 percent of respondents were veterans, as compared to 8 percent in the general U.S. population, and 0.5 percent were on active duty and 2 percent were in the National Guard or Reserves.

Among those currently serving in the military, 52 percent said they believed no one in the military knew of their transgender status, while 23 percent said a few knew, 22 percent that some knew, 8 percent that most knew, and 5 percent that everyone knew. Among those whose commanding officer knew of their status, 47 percent said the officer was supporting their desire to change their name and 36 percent supported their seeking medical treatment, while only 23 percent reported that their commanding officer took actions to discharge them.

Many veterans seek health care through the Veterans Administration (VA) system, and access to this system is an important benefit of military service. Of those who revealed their transgender status to their VA health-care provider, only 3 percent reported they were never treated respectfully due to their status. In contrast, 47 percent said they were always treated respectfully, 40 percent mostly respectfully, and 11 percent sometimes respectfully.

Agnes Gereben Schaefer and colleagues, in a 2016 study for the RAND Institute, estimate the number of transgender individuals currently serving in the American military as between 1,320 and 6,630, with a mid-range estimate of 2,450 transgender personnel. They estimate that only a subset of these service members will ever seek treatment related to gender transition, with an average of between 29 and 129 seeking gender transition-related care each year. Schaefer and colleagues estimate that, if transition-related care were available to all military personnel, the costs would be relatively low, with an increase of 0.04 to 0.13 percent increase in overall healthcare costs (the high-end estimate is just over one-tenth of 1%), and that less than 0.1 percent (one-tenth of 1%) would seek transition-related care that would interfere with their ability to deploy. They find no evidence from a study of foreign military organizations that integrating transgender individuals and offering them appropriate care has a negative impact on unit cohesion, operational effectiveness, or military readiness, and note commanders had stated that transgender-inclusive policies had the benefit of creating a more diverse and inclusive military force.

VIOLENCE AND HATE CRIMES
United States

Data from the 2015 U.S. Transgender Survey indicates that a substantial proportion of transgender individuals have experienced a physical attack within the past year. Overall, 13 percent of respondents reported at least one such experience in the past year. Of those who experienced such an attack, 66 percent identified gender identity or expression as the reason for the attack, with 32 percent reporting sexual orientation as the cause (victims could indicate more than one cause). Among those who were physically attacked, 45 percent report one such attack, 24 percent two attacks, 13 percent three attacks, and 16 percent four or more attacks.

Among those who had been attacked, the most common types of attack reported were being grabbed, punched, or choked (73%), having something (like a rock or a bottle) thrown at them (29%), and being sexually assaulted (29%); note that individuals could indicate more than one type of attack. Some subgroups were far more likely to have been attacked, including individuals working in the underground economy (41%), undocumented immigrants (24%), and those identifying as Middle Eastern (25%), or multiracial (19%).

Almost half (47%) of respondents reported being sexually assaulted at least once in their lives, with sexual assault much more common in some subgroups. Seventy-two percent of respondents who had engaged in sex work reported being sexually assaulted, as did 65 percent of those who had even been homeless and 61 percent of individuals with disabilities. Transgender men (51%) were more likely to have been sexually assaulted than transgender women (37%), while among racial and ethnic groups, American Indians (71%), Middle Eastern individuals (67%), and multiracial individuals (58%) reported the highest levels of sexual assault. The most common perpetrators of sexual assault were a friend or acquaintance (47%), a partner or ex-partner (34%), a stranger (30%), or a relative (25%).

Intimate partner violence (IPV) was also a common experience among respondents. Over half (54%) reported some lifetime experience with IPV, with higher rates among those who had done sex work (77%), had been homeless (72%), were undocumented (68%), had a disability (61%), or who identified as American Indian (73%), multiracial 62%), or Middle Eastern (62%). Forty-four percent of respondents reported experiencing a specific type of IPV, called "coercive control"; the most common behaviors reported included the partner telling them they were not a "real" man or woman (25%), trying to keep them apart from family or friends (23%), being stalked (16%), and being kept from leaving the house when they wanted to leave (15%). Forty-two percent reported experiencing physical violence resulting in harm from a partner, including being pushed or shoved (30%), being slapped (24%), forced to engage in sexual activity (19%), being hit with a fist or something hard (16%), and being slammed against something (14%). The rate of physical violence involving harm was highest among those identifying as American Indian (61%), multiracial (54%), or Middle Eastern (49%).

A hate crime is a type of bias crime in which the victim is targeted because of his or her characteristics, such as race, religion, or sexual or gender identity. James Comey, then director of the FBI, noted in a 2014 speech to the Anti-Defamation League National Leadership Summit that hate crimes are particularly insidious because they strike at the heart of the victim's identity, attacking their sense of self and belonging. The first U.S. law dealing with hate crimes was the Civil Rights Act of 1968, which defined hate crimes as attacks on individuals or their property related to their race, religion, or national origin. Mandatory annual reporting on hate crimes began with the Hate Crime Statistics Act of 1990 and hate crime statistics have been published by the FBI since 1996. However, the FBI has only included hate crimes motivated by gender or gender identification in these statistics since 2013.

Hate crime statistics should be interpreted with caution, because classifying a crime as a hate crime is in part a matter of judgment, and reporting may differ across different regions of the country. In addition, crimes may remain unreported, and this may also differ based on many factors. However, the FBI hate crimes report for 2015 (the most current year available) provides much useful information about this type of crime. In 2015, 6,837 single-bias (crimes motivated by a single bias, a category that includes most hate crimes) hate crime offenses were reported. Of those, 17.8 percent were motivated by bias against the victim's sexual identity (1,219 offenses), and 1.7 percent (118 offenses) by the victim's gender identity. Among the sexual-orientation bias offences, 62.2 percent were classified as anti-gay male, 19.3 as mixed group bias (anti-lesbian, gay, bisexual, or transgender), 13.8 percent as anti-lesbian bias, 2.9 percent as anti-bisexual bias, and 1.9 percent as anti-heterosexual bias. Among the offenses due to gender identity bias, 64 percent were due to anti-transgender bias and the remainder to anti-gender nonconforming bias.

Europe

Violence, and the threat of violence, are common experiences for many transgender people in Europe. Among transgender respondents to the 2014 European Union Lesbian, Gay, Bisexual and Transgender Survey, more than one-third (34%) said they had been physically or sexually attacked or threatened with violence in the past five years, and 15 percent reporting that they had had at least one such experience in the past year. Both percentages are noticeably higher even than for the other sexual minorities (lesbians, gay men, and bisexuals) included in this survey. Overall, 23 percent of the total sample reported being physically or sexually attacked or threatened with violence in the past five years, and 9 percent reporting that they had had at least one such experience in the past year.

Of those transgender respondents who had suffered at least one incident of violence in the past 12 months, 55 percent said they thought the last such incident was based on their transgender status. Such hate crimes were more commonly experienced by individuals whose birth sex and gender expression do not match (11%) than among those for which they do match (5%). The rate of violent incidents experienced in the past year by transgender individuals, 512 per 1,000 respondents, was almost twice as high for the sample as a whole (262 per 1,000 respondents). This indicates that even compared to other sexual minorities, transgender people are disproportionately the victims of violence. Of those who experienced at least one hate crime in the past year, 37 percent said the most recent incident was a threat of physical violence, 27 percent a physical attack, 17 percent a threat of both physical and sexual violence, 7 percent a physical and sexual attack, 5 percent a sexual attack, 2 percent a threat of sexual violence, and 1 percent did not know how to classify the most recent attack. Of those who suffered one or more hate crimes, only 24 percent of transgender respondents said they reported the most serious crime to the police.

PRISON AND THE CRIMINAL JUSTICE SYSTEM

Transgender people have high levels of contact with law enforcement, according to the results of the 2015 U.S. Transgender Survey. Forty percent of respondents said they interacted with law enforcement in the past year; of those individuals, 35 percent said they believed that some or all of the law enforcement officials they interacted believed they were transgender. Those who interact with law enforcement officials who knew or thought they were transgender report relatively high levels of respect, as 43 percent say they were always treated with respect, 43 percent that they were sometimes treated with respect, and 14 percent that they were never treated with respect. Those working in the underground economy were less likely to say that they were always treated with respect (20%), as were those living in poverty (31%), and those who were American Indian (28%) or black (30%).

Fifty-eight percent of those who believed the police officers interacting with them knew they were transgender reported at least one negative experience, the most common being the use of wrong titles (e.g., Mr. vs. Mrs.) or pronouns (49%), being verbally harassed (20%), and being asked about their gender transition when it was irrelevant (19%). Less commonly reported experiences include having the police assume they were sex workers (11%), being physically attacked (4%) or sexually assaulted (3%) by police officers, and being forced to engage in sexual activity to avoid arrest (1%). Negative experiences were more common among the homeless (78%) and unemployed (75%), among people with disabilities (68%), and among American Indians (74%), multiracial individuals (71%), Hispanics (65%), and blacks (61%).

Given this history of mistreatment, it may not be surprising that only 12 percent of respondents said they be very comfortable asking the police for help, and an additional 17 percent somewhat comfortable. In contrast, 31 percent said they would be very uncomfortable and 26 percent somewhat uncomfortable contacting the police for help, with 15 percent being neutral on this issue. The highest levels of discomfort (somewhat or very uncomfortable asking the police for help) occurred among people with disabilities (70%), those living in poverty (67%), those of Middle Eastern ethnicity (70%), and black and multiracial individuals (67% each).

Two percent of respondents were incarcerated (held in jail, prison, or a juvenile detention facility) in the past year, with higher rates of incarceration among undocumented individuals (12%), those who had been homeless in the past year (7%), and black transgender women (9%). Among those who had been incarcerated in the past year, 20 percent reported being sexually assaulted by staff or other inmates, five to six times higher than is reported among the total population of those who are incarcerated. Fifty-eight percent of respondents who were incarcerated had been taking hormones at the time, with 82 percent of those taking hormones having a prescription for them. However, many could not continue hormone therapy while in jail, with over one-third (37%) of those taking hormones at the time of their incarceration being prohibited from continuing to take their hormones while incarcerated.

Among respondents who were not American citizens, 4 percent said they had been in immigration detention at least once in their lifetime. Among those held in immigration, 45 percent report mistreatment or assault, including 29 percent reporting they were denied access to hormones, 23 percent physical assault, 22 percent being denied gender-appropriate clothing, 19 percent threats of sexual assault, and 15 percent experiencing sexual assault.

CREDENTIALING

Official identification or credentials, such as a passport or driver's license, generally includes not only a person's name but also their sex or gender. While there are usually official procedures in place to allow a person to change their name on such identification (e.g., due to a marriage or a legal name change), transgender individuals who wish to change their designated sex (e.g., from male to female or female to male) often encounter obstacles in obtaining credentials reflecting their new status.

This is a problem because such identification is required for many functions of life, from getting a job to boarding an airplane to enrolling in school. Transgender people also face barriers in getting their name and/or sex changed on official records such as school transcripts or military discharge papers, making it difficult for them to present such credentials in support of employment applications or other procedures.

United States

A report published in 2016 by the National Center for Transgender Equality, written by Sandy E. James and colleagues, found that many American transgender people have experienced difficulty in obtaining credentials reflecting their preferred name and gender identity. This is reflected in the fact that only 11 percent of the sample studied reported that all their records and IDs reflected both their preferred name and gender identity, while 67 percent did not have even one ID or record reflecting their preferred gender, and 49 percent did not have even one ID or record carrying their preferred name.

The procedures for obtaining a legal name change, which is usually a prerequisite for obtaining a name change on ID or records, is established at the state or territorial level, so the experience of requesting such a change depends in part on where an individual lives. About one-third (36%) of respondents reported attempting to change their name legally, with 30 percent succeeding in doing so. Most (60%) who attempted to change their name said they did so without assistance, while 17 percent reported receiving help from a legal clinic or nonprofit operation, 11 percent help from a friend, 9 percent help from a paid attorney, and 7 percent help from another source.

For those who did not attempt a legal name change, some felt they were simply not ready for the change (40%) or that there was no conflict between their current name and their gender identity or expression (28%). Others reported facing barriers such as cost (35%), lack of information about how to go about it (24%), fear of revealing their transgender status (24%), or not knowing that such a change was possible (3%); respondents were allowed to select more than one reason, so the percentages add up to more than 100 percent. The cost associated with obtaining a legal name change varied broadly among respondents, with 7 percent reporting that they incurred no costs, and 1 percent saying it cost over $2,000. Over half (55%) reported a cost between $100 and $499, 20 percent a cost between $1 and $99, and 10 percent a cost between $500 and $2,000 (8% said they did not remember how much it cost).

Two-thirds of the respondents did not have any ID or records listing their preferred gender, while only 12 percent had their preferred gender on all their IDs and records. The procedure to change one's gender on official documents varies by state but often requires the individual to present supporting documentation such as a court order of gender change or documentation by a healthcare provider of a gender change. Among those who had a particular type of identification or record and wanted to change their gender on it, the greatest number had changed their gender on their driver's license or state nondriver ID (29%), followed by their social security records (23%), passport (18%), records for last school attended (18%), and birth certificate (9%). Success rates in changing the gender designation varied by the type of ID or record, with the greatest success (90%) among those who sought to change their driver's license, followed by social security records (70%), passport (55%), student records at last school attended (55%), and birth certificate (27%).

There was considerable diversity within the sample regarding the choice to change one's gender designation on an official ID or record, with those who had transitioned and identified as transgender most likely to have made the change. For instance, 52 percent of those who had transitioned and identified as transgender had updated their driver's license to reflect their new gender, as compared to 42 percent among all who had transitioned, and 9 percent of those who had transitioned and identified their gender as nonbinary (i.e., neither male nor female). Similar patterns were seen for other types of ID; for instance, for social security records, 52 percent of people who had transitioned and identified as transgender had changed the sex designation on their records, as compared to 33 percent among everyone who had transitioned, 23 percent of the total sample, and 4 percent of those who had transitioned and identified as nonbinary.

Many transgender people do not have identification that matches their preferred name and gender, and almost one-third (32%) reported negative experiences when using such an ID, including being attacked, harassed, or refused services. Overall, 25 percent of the sample reported being verbally harassed, with this experience varying by race and ethnicity. The highest rates of verbal harassment after presenting an ID with a name and/or gender that did not match the individual's gender presentation being Middle Eastern (44%) or American Indian (39%), as compared to 33 percent of multiracial individuals, Hispanics (27%), blacks (24%), and whites (24%). Similarly, only 2 percent reported being assaulted, but the percentage was higher for Middle Eastern people (9%), followed by American Indians (6%), blacks (4%), Asians (3%), multiracial people (3%), Hispanics (2%), and whites (2%).

Canada

In Canada, procedures for changing one's gender designation on official documents are established separately for each province. For instance, to change the gender designation on one's birth certificate in Ontario, an individual must be at least 18 years old and have been born in Ontario. There is no requirement (as was formerly the case) to have undergone sexual reassignment surgery, but the individual must provide a number of forms and documents, including all previous birth certificates and a letter from a physician, psychologist, or psychological associate indicating that they have treated the individual in question, that individual's gender identity does not correspond with the sex designation on the birth certificate, and that changing the sex designation on the birth certificate is appropriate. Ontario also has procedures in place to allow an individual to change his or her gender designation on his or her driver's license and provincial health insurance card.

Credentialing proved difficult for many respondents of a 2015 report by Greta Bauer and Aydem I. Scheim, which analyzes data from several Trans PULSE surveys of transgender people in Ontario. For the respondents to these surveys who had changed their legal names and were living in a gender different from the one they were classified as at birth, 31 percent reporting not having changed their identity documents (e.g., passport, driver's license, health card) to reflect their new status. A much higher percentage, 58 percent, reported they could not get academic transcripts with their correct name and pronoun.

As of July 2016, the Canadian government was considering allowing gender-neutral designations on official IDs and documents in order to accommodate those whose gender identity does not correspond to the male/female binary system. The province of Ontario had already instituted such a system for driver's licenses, allowing individuals to designate their gender as "X" rather than male or female; some other countries, including Australia and New Zealand also allow individuals to designate their gender as "X" rather than male or female.

Europe

In 1992, the European Court of Human Rights declared that it was a violation of the European Convention on Human Rights for a country to refuse to allow transgender people to change their gender designation on official documents. However, as of 2017, some countries under the jurisdiction of the European Court of Human Rights (47 countries, including most of Europe except for Poland, plus Turkey) still do not allow individuals to change their gender designation, while others require individuals to undergo a lengthy process that may include getting an official diagnosis of a mental disorder and undergoing hormonal and/or surgical treatments before they are allowed to change their gender designation. Such requirements mean that a transgender person must give up some of their human rights, including the right to reproduce, in order to have their felt gender recognized by the state. Some also impose age requirements or require that an individual be unmarried before undertaking such a change.

Among transgender respondents to the 2014 European Union Lesbian, Gay, Bisexual and Transgender Survey, 5 percent said they could change official documents in their country of residence to match their preferred gender without having to meet any obligatory criteria, 67 percent said they could make such changes after meeting obligatory criteria, 9 percent said they could not, and 19 percent were not sure.

A 2014 report by Amnesty International examined the current status of transgender rights in seven high-income European countries: Denmark, Finland, France, Ireland, Norway, Belgium, and Germany. This report found that, despite the 1992 decision by the European Court of Human Rights that individuals should be able to change gender markers on their official documents, legal implementation of this right is far from complete and often comes with invasive and arduous requirements—for instance, an individual may be required to undergo surgical or hormonal treatments before being allowed to change his or her gender markers on official documents.

Since 2014, some of the countries included in this report have reformed the process by which an individual may change his or her gender identity on official documents. For instance, in Denmark, an individual aged 18 or over can simply request new official documents, without requiring a statement from a medical or psychiatric expert, and without undergoing any specific medical procedures; the primary requirement is a six-month waiting period before the change takes effect. In contrast, as of 2017, Finland still required trans people to undergo sterilization before they can change their gender identity on official documents and records. Laws regarding transgender people are changing rapidly in many countries, so this is one area where it is advisable to check the latest available information before making statements about the current situation in any specific country.

PUBLIC SPACES

Independent of specific consequences of discrimination (e.g., being refused a job based on one's transgender status), many transgender people avoid public spaces such as parks, malls, or restaurants because they want to avoid being harassed or attacked. This limits the ability of transgender people to take part in public life and to be a full member of the community in which they live and prevents them from enjoying the same choices and opportunities available to other members of their community.

United States

About one-third (31%) of respondents to the 2015 U.S. Transgender Survey report a negative experience in a public place within the past year due to their transgender status. The most common experience was verbal harassment (24%), followed by denial of equal treatment or service (14%), and physical attack (2%) (respondents could indicate more than one category).

Two percent of respondents reported they did not use public transportation in the past year because of fear of harassment; among those who did use public transportation and who believed employees knew or believed they were harassment, 34 percent reported one or more negative experiences, most often verbal harassment (32%), with smaller numbers reporting denial of equal treatment or service (4%) or physical attack (3%). Those living in poverty (39%) were more likely to report negative experiences on public transportation, as were those working in the underground economy (49%). Among racial and ethnic groups, American Indians were most likely to have a negative experience (48%), followed by multiracial individuals (45%) and Asians (39%).

Most (91%) of respondents indicated visiting a retail store, restaurant, hotel, or theatre in the past year, with only 1 percent reporting avoiding such locations due to fear of mistreatment. Of those who had visited one more such locations, and who believed staff knew or thought they were transgender, 31 percent report one or more negative experiences due to their status. Most common among these experiences was verbal harassment (24%), followed by denial of equal treatment or service (11%), and physical attack (1%). Negative experiences were most common among those working in the underground economy (52%), and among American Indian (49%) and multiracial (41%) individuals.

More than one-third (35%) of respondents had visited a gym or health club in the past year, while 14 percent had avoided such places out of fear of mistreatment. Of those who had visited a gym or health club and believed staff or employees knew or believed they were transgender, 18 percent reported one or more negative experiences. Verbal harassment (13%) was the most common, followed by denial of equal treatment or service (7%), and physical attack (1%).

Twelve percent of respondents had visited a government benefits or public assistance office in the past year, while 2 percent avoided visiting such places due to fear of mistreatment. Of those who visited such offices and believed staff knew or believed they were transgender, 17 percent report negative experiences, including denial of equal treatment or service (11%) and verbal harassment (9%). Negative experiences were most common among those who worked in the underground economy (24%), had disabilities (21%), or were American Indian (25%), multiracial (22%), or black or Hispanic (each 20%).

Over half (53%) of respondents reported going through airport security in the past year. Of those, 43 percent reported having at least one issue due to their gender identity or expression. The most common experience was being addressed by incorrect pronouns or title (29%), followed by being patted down due to gender-related clothing (e.g., a chest binder) (17%), and being patted down by a TSA employee of the wrong gender (14%). Other negative experiences included having a TSA employee loudly refer to or question their gender or referring to items such as a binder (6%), having their bag searched due to containing items such as a binder (5%), and being asked to remove or lift clothing to display a usually concealed part of their body or clothing (4%).

Canada

A 2011 survey of 433 individuals age 16 or older who live, work, or receive health care in Ontario, conducted by TRANS Pulse, found that about two-thirds of respondents avoided public places or situations out of fear of harassment or because they did not want to be publicly identified as transgender. This experience was even more common for those who had begun to live in their felt gender, with 83 percent reporting such avoidance, and among those who had experienced violence due to their transgender status, with almost all (97%) individuals reporting some avoidance of public situations. Public facilities that transgender people reported avoiding due to their status included schools, restaurants, malls, gyms, and public restrooms.

Europe

Many transgender people in Europe suffer from discrimination when accessing ordinary services and places of business, according to the European Union Lesbian, Gay, Bisexual and Transgender Survey. Nineteen percent said they had experienced discrimination on the basis of their status in a café, bar, or restaurant, 17 percent in a shop, 10 percent in a bank or insurance office, and 15 percent in a sport or fitness club. These levels were generally higher than for the other sexual minorities included in the survey, with 18 percent of the total sample reporting discrimination in a café, bar, or restaurant, 8 percent in a shop, 4 percent in a bank or insurance office, and 15 percent in a sport or fitness club.

Transgender respondents to the survey report high levels of harassment, with over half (58%) saying that they were harassed by a person or group in the past five years, and 35 percent having such an experience in the past year. Harassment can include a variety of behaviors, including name calling, ridiculing, bullying, and aggressive gestures. These levels are the highest for any of the sexual minorities included in the European Union Lesbian, Gay, Bisexual and Transgender Survey (the survey also includes lesbian, gay, and bisexual individuals), and higher than the overall average of 47 percent who had been harassed in the past five years, and 25 percent who had been harassed in the past year. The incidence rate of harassment (the number of incidents relative to population) was also higher for transgender individuals, with 1,753 incidents per 1,000 respondents (i.e., on average almost two per respondent), as compared to 1,012 per 1,000 for the sample as a whole.

Another measure of harassment is how often individuals feel it necessary to modify their behavior in public to avoid assault or harassment. For instance, 58 percent of transgender respondents to the European Union Lesbian, Gay, Bisexual and Transgender Survey said they avoided holding hands with their partner in public to avoid assault or harassment, and 32 percent said they avoided expressing their gender identity by their clothing and physical appearance out of fear of assault or harassment. Fifty percent said they avoided certain places or locations due to fear of harassment.

CHAPTER 7

Access to Health and Social Services and Public Facilities

Transgender people face many barriers in accessing health and social services and public facilities. In the United States, transgender people are more likely than the general population to be uninsured, and even those with insurance may face barriers to receiving optimal health care, both for transition-related issues and for health concerns having nothing to do with their transgender status. Transgender people also face barriers accessing social benefits, such as subsidized housing, and may be subject to legally mandated discrimination with regard to their use of public restrooms and other sex-segregated facilities.

HEALTH INSURANCE

Transgender individuals in the United States are somewhat more likely than the general population to be uninsured, according to a 2016 report by Sandy E. James and colleagues based on the 2015 U.S. Transgender Survey. Fourteen percent of respondents to the survey reported they were uninsured, as compared to 11 percent of adults in the entire U.S. population. Transgender people living in the South were most likely to be uninsured (20%), as compared to those in the Midwest (13%), West (11%), or Northeast (9%). The rate of uninsurance also varied by race and ethnicity, with blacks (20%), American Indians (18%), multiracial individuals (16%), while those who were white (12%), Asian (11%) or Middle Eastern (11%) were less likely to be uninsured. Immigration status was also related to insurance status, with over half (58%) of undocumented respondents and almost a quarter (24%) of documented noncitizen respondents lacking health insurance.

Many respondents reported experiencing problems with their insurer in the past year based on their transgender status. The most common complain were being refused coverage for surgery related to their transition (55% of those who made such a request) and receiving only partial coverage for surgery related to their transition (42%). Other problems reported including being denied coverage for hormones related to their transition (25%), being unable to find a surgical provider within the insurer's network to perform transition-related surgery (21%), being unable to change their name and/or gender in the insurer's records (17%), being denied gender-specific care because of their transgender status (13%), and being denied other routine health care because of their transgender status (7%) (note that individuals could indicate more than one problem, so percentages total more than 100).

There was some variation in denial of care based on the type of insurance the respondent held. The highest rates of denial of coverage for hormone therapy in the past year was experienced by those covered only by Medicaid (29%) or only by private insurance (26%), with lower rates of denial for those covered by multiple types of insurance (21%), other types of insurance (20%), or Medicare only (14%). There was less variation in the rate of refusal for transgender surgery, except for a lower rate of refusal for Medicare: 55 percent of those with Medicaid only, private insurance only, and other insurance only reported such a refusal in the past year, as compared to 54 percent of those with multiple types of insurance, and 48 percent for those with Medicare only.

Gender differences were also observed in the rates of refusal for transgender-related care. Transgender women and nonbinary individuals designated as male on their original birth certificate experienced lower rates of refusal for hormone treatments (18% and 16%, respectively) than did transgender men (32%) and nonbinary people designated as female on their original birth certificate (36%). A similar pattern was present in refusals for transgender surgery: transgender women and those designated as male on their original birth certificate experienced refusal rates of 54 percent and 35 percent, respectively, as compared to refusal rates of 57 percent for transgender men and 54 percent for nonbinary people designated as female on their original birth certificate.

Canada

Although Canada provides universal, publicly funded health care, the healthcare system is administered separately in each province or territory within guidelines set by the federal government. This means that the availability of services may vary from one province or territory to another, including some transgender health care. As of 2016, all provinces provided some care for transgender-related surgery, but which specific surgeries are covered varies by province, as does the distance a person might have to travel to receive transgender-related surgery. Of the territories, only the Yukon provides coverage for transgender-related surgery, while Nunavut and the Northwest Territories do not.

Coverage varies by gender—for instance, trans men are covered for mastectomy in all provinces, but no provinces covered breast reconstruction for trans women. Quebec covers the most transgender-related surgical procedures, and all are performed within the province, with the Centre Metropolitain de Chirurgie (Metropolitan Surgical Center) in Montreal providing specific procedures for some individuals from other provinces as well (the individual's home province pays for the care). For instance, patients requiring more advanced care such as vaginoplasty may be referred to the Centre Metropolitain de Chirurgie because no surgeon in their home province is available to that procedure. As of 2018, Canada has two centers providing transgender-related surgery. The limited number of sites providing transgender-related surgery means that some individuals must wait years before they receive surgery for which they have been approved.

Barriers to Health Care

A 2011 report by the Institute of Medicine found that sexual and gender minorities, including transgender people, face many barriers when in accessing health care. Some of those barriers are directly related to an individual's sexual or gender status, others to characteristics such as income level, racial or ethnic minority status, and multiple factors can work together to impair access to health care. These factors may result in *stigma*, a term describing the inferior status assigned to some groups in a society. Along with inferior status, individuals identified as belonging to such groups may also suffer from the negative regard of others and from relative powerlessness within the society.

Stigma may be expressed in various ways, with three being particularly relevant to health care: enacted stigma, felt stigma, and internalized stigma. *Enacted stigma* refers to overt behaviors by others toward the stigmatized group, such as taunting, shunning, or physical attack. In terms of health care, enacted stigma could range from disrespectful behavior based on an individual's declared or perceived gender or sexual identity to refusal of treatment or provision of inferior treatment. *Felt stigma* refers to an individual's understanding that they may be treated badly due to some aspect of themselves, such as their gender or sexual identity. Felt stigma may cause an individual to fail to disclose some aspect of their lives, such as their sexual behavior, resulting in a medical record that is less than complete, and may also result in an individual not seeking health care when they should.

Internalized stigma refers to an individual accepting a societally approved negative view of some group, such as transgender people. Healthcare providers who have internalized stigmas regarding sexual and gender minorities may be uncomfortable in providing care to such individuals, and even if they try to hide their feelings they may betray them unconsciously to a patient. Internalized stigma can also apply to members of disadvantaged groups, so that, for instance, a transgender person may accept negative societal views of their own transgender status. Besides the shame such an individual may feel, internalized stigma may also cause them to avoid the healthcare system altogether, fail to disclose their status, and/or fail to challenge mistreatment based on their status.

Another barrier to seeking care is an experience of poor treatment from a medical provider based on one's gender identity. Most (87%) of respondents to the 2015 National Transgender Survey had seen a healthcare provider in the past year, but 33 percent reported having one or more negative experiences due to their transgender status. The most common experience was having to educate the provider about transgender people (24%), being asked invasive or unnecessary questions not related to the reason they were seeking care (15%), being refused care for a transition-related condition (8%), being verbally harassed in a healthcare setting (6%), being addressed harshly or abusively by a healthcare provider (5%), being refused routine care not related to transition (3%), a provider being physically rough or abusive (2%), being physically attacked at a healthcare setting (1%) and being sexually assaulted in a healthcare setting (1%). Perhaps because of the prevalence of such negative experiences, nearly one-third (31%) of respondents said they had not revealed their transgender status to any of the healthcare providers, while only 40 percent reported that all their current providers knew of their status.

The rate of such negative experiences varied by race and ethnicity, gender identity, and disability status. The highest percentage of respondents in any racial or ethnic group reporting at least one negative experience occurred among American Indians (50%) and was lowest among Asians (26%), with 40 percent of Middle Eastern individuals reporting such experiences, along with 38 percent of multiracial individuals, 34 percent each of black and white individuals, and 32 percent of Hispanic individuals. The rate of negative experiences was highest among transgender men

(42%), followed by transgender women (36%) and nonbinary individuals (24%). Negative experiences were also more common among people with a disability (42%) than with those not having a disability (30%).

Survey respondents reported a number of other barriers to receiving health care. The most common reason for foregoing necessary care was cost (33%), with this reason cited more often by people with disabilities (42%), multiracial individuals (42%), American Indians (41%), blacks (40%), and Latinos (37%), and less often by whites (31%) and Asians (27%). Another common reason for not seeking health care, reported by 23 percent of respondents, was fear of mistreatment due to transgender status. This reason was cited by 37 percent of American Indians, 34 percent of Middle Eastern people, 28 percent of multiracial people, 26 percent each of blacks and Hispanics, 24 percent of Asians, and 22 percent of white. It was also cited by a higher percentage of transgender men (31%) than transgender women (22%) and nonbinary individuals (20%).

Many respondents reported having to travel further to receive transition-related health care than to receive routine health care. For instance, 63 percent of respondents said they traveled less than 10 miles to receive routine health care, but only 45 percent said that they traveled 10 miles or less to receive transition-related care. In contrast, 12 percent said they traveled 50 miles or more to receive transition-related health care, while only 5 percent said they traveled that far to receive routine health care.

Canada

Among respondents to the Canadian Trans Youth Health Survey, over 70 percent reported having a family doctor, and over half of those (53%) reported that their family doctor knew about their trans identity. However, only 15 percent reported feeling very comfortable in discussing trans-related health care with their family doctor, while 27 percent felt comfortable, 30 percent uncomfortable, and 27 percent very uncomfortable. Respondents reported much less comfort in dealing with physicians at walk-in clinics: only 4 percent said they felt very comfortable discussing trans-related health care with such physicians, while 18 percent reported feeling comfortable, 40 percent uncomfortable, and 37 percent very uncomfortable.

Many respondents perceived that they had been the target of unprofessional behavior from physicians or other healthcare professionals based on their transgender status. For instance, 21 percent reported avoiding using the emergency room when they felt they needed care, due to fear of discrimination or harassment. These fears seem to be well-founded, as

25 percent said an emergency care provider had in fact ridiculed or belittled their transgender status, and 10 percent of those who sought care in an emergency room felt they had been refused care or had care terminated prematurely based on their status. For respondents who had a family physician, about 40 percent said that they had been discriminated against by that physician at least once; examples of such discrimination include being ridiculed or addressed in demeaning language, or being refused care or being refused examination of specific body parts.

One-third of younger trans youth (aged 14–18) reported that they had not received needed health care at some point in the past year, as did almost half (47%) of older trans youth (aged 19–25). The most common reasons for not accessing medical care when needed, among young trans youth (the question was not asked of older trans youth), were thinking or hoping the problem would go away (71%), being afraid of what the doctor might say or do (61%), didn't want parents to know (49%), being too busy (36%), not knowing where to go (35%), and having previous negative experiences (34%).

Europe

Almost one-fifth (19%) of transgender respondents to the 2014 European Union Lesbian, Gay, Bisexual and Transgender Survey reported being discriminated against by healthcare personnel in the past 12 months due to their status, almost twice the percentage (10%) reported by the total sample (which included, gay, lesbian, and bisexual people as well). The most common complaints reported by transgender people included inappropriate curiosity (21%; note that this question asked for experiences over a person's lifetime, not just the past year), specific needs being ignored (17%), being forced or pressured into taking some medical or psychological test (15%), foregoing treatment due to fears of discrimination or intolerance (14%), having to change general practitioners due to negative reaction (12%), difficulty in gaining access to health care (12%), and receiving unequal treatment from medical staff (11%).

RECOMMENDATIONS FOR HEALTHCARE PROFESSIONALS

One reason many transgender people experience mistreatment in the healthcare system may be that even the most well-meaning medical professionals may be as confused and uninformed about transgender people as the general public, and thus may unintentionally act in ways that might be experienced as offensive or harmful. To help remediate this situation, various guidelines have been published by transgender groups that seek to inform medical professionals and others involved in health care and health policy about transgender people and appropriate ways to treat them.

Guidelines for the Primary and Gender-Affirming Care of Transgender and Gender Nonbinary People, edited by Madeline B. Deutsch and published by the Center of Excellence for Transgender Health at the University of California, San Francisco, was written to help primary care providers and health systems meet the needs of transgender and gender-nonconforming individuals. These guidelines begin with advice on creating a safe and welcoming environment for transgender individuals, discussing special considerations when conducting vaginal exams with transgender women and pelvic exams with transgender men, and provide an overview of gender-affirming treatments and procedures. This document then provides details of many aspects of transgender health care, from hormone therapy to particular considerations for transgender individuals with regards to common diseases such as diabetes and cardiovascular disease and screening procedures for diseases such as breast cancer and osteoporosis.

These guidelines provide a wealth of concrete information for providers, including highly specific information relevant to transgender patients. It also provides a general approach to transgender care that is relevant in many other contexts. One major recommendation is that providers adopt an attitude of cultural humility, becoming aware of their own experiences and identities without assuming they apply to others, and thus approaching each patient as an individual and without preconceptions. They recommend training be provided to all staff members who interact with patients (e.g., those working at intake desks), that the waiting areas include transgender-themed materials to indicate that transgender people are welcome, that at least one restroom be gender-neutral and individuals be allowed to use the restroom of their choice, and that providers and other staff familiarize themselves with terminology used in the transgender community.

They suggest gender information be collected in two steps: first, the individual's gender identity (e.g., male, female, trans man, trans woman, genderqueer), and second, the sex assigned at birth (male or female), allowing the individual to decline to answer either question if that is their preference. They also recommend collecting data about preferred name and pronoun upon intake, and recommend that the electronic medical records systems used by many healthcare organizations be revised to accommodate collecting and recording such information.

Jennifer Potter and colleagues issued guidelines for physicians on providing cervical cancer screening to female-to-male transgender people.
They begin by establishing the need for such guidelines, citing a survey
that found that 11 percent of obstetrician-gynecologists were unwilling
to provide routine Pap tests for transgender patients, and only 29 percent
felt comfortable caring for female-to-male individuals. This is a problem,
because Pap tests, also called Pap smears, are part of routine cervical cancer screening for women and are medically indicated for adults who have
a cervix, regardless of their gender presentation. In addition, transgender individuals have been shown to be less likely to be up-to-date on Pap
smears than the general population, possibly in part due to anticipated
insensitivity from healthcare providers not accustomed to treating transgender people.

The recommendations of Potter and colleagues begin with common-
sense suggestions such as asking a patient for their preferred name and
pronouns and using them through the clinical encounter. They recommend
reviewing the procedure with the patient, describing it as a method of cancer screening rather than a screening specific to the female reproductive
system. They also recommend use of nongendered language whenever
possible, for example, referring to underwear rather than bra and panties,
and avoid violent or sexual language (e.g., "let your legs drop to either
side" rather than "open your legs").

Transgender-Affirming Hospital Policies, written by Lambda Legal
in conjunction with the Human Rights Campaign Foundation, Hogan
Lovells, and the New York City Bar, proposes seven model policies that
hospitals may adopt to protect the rights of transgender people. This document includes both the language of the proposed policies, and explanation
of why each policy is important.

The first two model policies extend hospital statements of nondis-
crimination, which typically cover categories such as race and religion,
to include gender identity and expression. First, the hospital nondiscrim-
ination policy should include the statement that no one will be discriminated against due to their gender expression or gender identity. Second,
the hospital's Patients' Bill of Right should include a statement that
patients have the right to care in a safe setting free of abuse or harassment based on gender identity or expression. The third policy states that
transgender patients should have access to hormone therapy if they have
been receiving it before admission, and that if a provider is unfamiliar
with hormone therapy, the provider should consult with other providers
who do have that expertise, including if possible the patient's prescribing physician.

The fourth policy states that hospital staff should treat transgender patients with courtesy and respect. This includes using appropriate name and pronouns (honoring the patient's view, even if family members have a different opinion), refraining from using language or tone that is demeaning or invalidating, and refraining from inquiring about an individual's sexual or other characteristics, or surgical status, unless such inquiries are medically necessary.

The fifth and sixth policies deal with the use of facilities that are assigned according to gender. The fifth policy states that if room assignments are based on gender, the patient's self-identified gender should be used for this purpose, with appropriate privacy assured by means such as assignment to a single room or the use of curtains within a room. The sixth policy states that transgender people should be able to use restrooms based on their gender identity, and should be protected from harassment while doing so. The seventh policy states that transgender people should have access to personal items that facilitate their gender expression, including clothing, makeup, and items used for purposes such as packing or binding, on the same basis as other patients.

This policy document also provides recommendations for administrative processes within the hospital, and staff training, that will facilitate the appropriate care of transsexual people. For instance, intake forms should collect information about both current identity and identity at birth, and information about current name in use as well as legal name. Staff members should be trained to collect this information in a sensitive manner, and to protect patients' privacy and treat every patient with respect and dignity.

ACCESS TO HOUSING

Home ownership is much less common among transgender individuals than the general U.S. population, according to the 2015 U.S. Transgender Survey. Overall, 16 percent of respondents owned their own home, as compared to 63 percent of the general population. Home ownership was lower in every age group among transgender individuals than in the general population, with the greatest differences seen in the younger age groups. For instance, only 11 percent of transgender people in the 25 to 24 age group owned their home, as compared to 37 percent of the general population in that age group. In contrast, among those 65 and older, 69 percent of transgender individuals owned their own home, as compared to 78 percent of the general population.

Thirty percent of respondents to the 2015 U.S. Transgender Survey reported being homeless at least once, with some subgroups experiencing much higher rates of homelessness. Among those who had been forced out of their immediate family's home, 74 percent report being homeless at some point in their lives; of those living with HIV, 59 percent have been homeless at least once, as have 59 percent of those who have done sex work and 55 percent of those who have lost their job due to their gender identity or expression. Twelve percent of respondents indicated experiencing homelessness due to their transgender status, with 6 percent reporting that they were denied a home or apartment in the past year due to their transgender status, and 5 percent reporting being kicked out of their home or apartment due to their transgender status.

Among respondents who had been homeless in the past year, 26 percent did not seek access to a homeless shelter because they feared mistreatment due to their transgender status, and 6 percent said they were denied access to one or more shelter. Asians (43%) and American Indians (37%) were more likely than average to avoid seeking access to a homeless shelter out of fear of mistreatment, as were those working in the underground economy (36%) or who had been kicked out of their family's home (35%). Among those who were denied access to at least one homeless shelter, 74 percent said they believed the reason for denial was their gender identity or expression.

Among those respondents who had stayed in at least one homeless shelter in the past year, 70 percent reported at least one negative experience at the shelter. Almost half (44%) said they left the shelter because of unsafe conditions or poor treatment, despite having no place to go to. One-quarter (25%) said they dressed or presented as the gender they did not identify with in order to feel safe, 14 percent said the shelter required such dress or presentation, and 9 percent said they were thrown out of the shelter when their transgender status was discovered. Over half (52%) said they were harassed, attacked, or assaulted while staying in a homeless shelter, with 49 percent reporting verbal harassment, 19 percent physical attack, and 17 percent sexual assault (respondents could report more than one type of experience).

Many respondents to the 2011 National Transgender Discrimination survey also reported difficulties in obtaining shelter housing. Fifty-five percent reported experiencing harassment by shelter staff or residents, 22 percent sexual assault by residents or staff, and 29 percent report being turned away from the shelter due to their transgender status. This is particularly relevant because many transgender people are also subject to other types of discrimination (including difficulties in finding employment, and rejection by family and friends), which may lead to them becoming homeless. Nineteen percent report being homeless due to their transgender at some point in their lives, with 11 percent reporting eviction due to their status and 19 percent having been refused a home or apartment because of their status.

ACCESS TO PUBLIC RESTROOMS

Many people are familiar with the difficulties transgender people may encounter when seeking to use a public restroom, because in the United States it is common to have separate facilities for men and women. Many states have recently introduced or passed legislation to require transgender people to use the restroom designated for the sex they were assigned at birth, regardless of their current gender identity; North Carolina was the first to pass such a law, in March 2016. Some institutions, including colleges and universities, have begun designating some restrooms as gender-free or otherwise indicating that they may be used without regard to an individual's sex or gender, and California law (as of March 1, 2017) requires that single-occupancy public restrooms be designated as gender neutral. However, this practice is far from universal, and many transgender people encounter difficulties in using public restroom facilities, particularly if their gender presentation does not match their sex assigned at birth.

Even before "bathroom bills" such as that passed in 2016 in North Carolina existed, many transgender people encountered violence or harassment when using public restrooms. Among respondents to the 2015 U.S. Transgender Survey, 24 percent said they had been questioned or told they were using the wrong restroom in the past year, and 9 percent said they were denied access to a restroom. Those working in the underground economy (20%) and undocumented individuals (23%) were even more likely to report having been denied access to a restroom, as were American Indians (18%), Asians (13%), Middle Eastern individuals (12%), multiracial individuals (11%), and Hispanics (10%).

One reason often given for denying transgender people the right to use the restroom of their choice is that they pose a danger to cisgender people, particularly women. However, reported assaults by transgender people in restrooms are extremely rare (one commentator noted that more Republican politicians have been arrested for sex crimes in restrooms than have transgender people for attacking others in restrooms). On the other hand, many transgender people have been the victims of crimes in restrooms, and an even higher number have been harassed, making the safety of transgender people in this context a serious issue.

Twelve percent of respondents to the 2015 U.S. Transgender Survey reported being verbally harassed, physically attacked, or sexually assaulted in the past year while using a public restroom, with such experiences even more common among undocumented people (34%), those working in the underground economy (25%), and among American Indians (24%) and individuals of mixed race (16%). Overall, 12 percent report verbal harassment, 1 percent physical attack, and 0.6 percent sexual assault in a restroom in the past year.

Over half (59%) of respondents report avoiding using a restroom in the past year due to fear of confrontation or some other difficulty, with such avoidance more common among transgender men (75%), undocumented individuals (72%), and those who said others could always or usually detect that they were transgender. Almost one-third reported that they avoided eating or drinking in some circumstances to avoid needing to use a public restroom.

CHAPTER 8

Transgender Athletes: Who Competes against Whom?

One of the most public areas of controversy involving transgender people has been that of participation in sports, in particular the participation of trans women on an equal basis with cisgender women in competitions. This chapter looks at the reasons why men and women often compete separately in sports, the problems posed by transgender people to an arrangement that recognizes only two genders, and offers a brief history of gender testing and trans women in sports. It also looks at how transgender athletes have been treated in school competitions and offers recommendations to make school sports more inclusive.

WHY IS GENDER CLASSIFICATION IMPORTANT IN SPORTS?

Many sports activities are organized so that men compete against men, and women against women. This classification is based on the average physical differences between adult men and women—men tend to be larger and stronger, for instance, while women are more flexible. These differences give men advantages in many popular sports, such as athletics (track and field), swimming, basketball, football (both American football and soccer), and tennis. Exceptions to the general rule of gender-separated teams and competitions include teams and competitions for children below the age of puberty (e.g., Little League baseball) and in sports the physical differences between adult men and women lend little or no advantage in competition (e.g., equestrian events). Recreational sports competitions, where the emphasis is on participation rather than elite competition, may also include male and female players on an equal basis, although coed sports often have rules governing how many men and women must be on a team to prevent teams from stacking the lineup with men. Some sports, such as gymnastics, are also structured differently for men and women. For instance, in gymnastics men compete on the pommel horse, still rings, parallel bars, and horizontal bars, women compete on the uneven bars and balance beam, and both men and women compete in the vault and floor exercise.

As Vanessa Heggie points out, organizing sports competitions separately for men and women implies that human beings come in only two sexual forms, male and female, and that one of those forms has significant biological advantages that would make competition between the two sexes inherently unequal. Because it is women who are generally perceived to be at a disadvantage relative to men in most sports, various tests have been devised to determine who qualifies as female.

There is no question that in many athletic endeavors, adult men hold significant advantages over adult women. To put this into perspective, consider the fact that the world record for men for the 100 meters is 9.58 seconds, set by Usain Bolt in 2009. The world record for women is 10.49 seconds, set by Florence Griffith-Joyner in 1988. Setting aside the fact that many believe Griffith-Joyner's record was wind-aided, the women's record is almost a full second slower than the male world record. In the 2016 Summer Olympics, the *slowest* male runner to advance out of the heats ran a time of 10.20, or more than a quarter second faster than the fastest time ever run by a woman. The last time Griffith-Joyner's time would have qualified as a men's world record was in 1912, and the American boy's high school record for the 100 meters, 10.00 seconds, is faster by almost half a second than her best time ever.

So, if men and women had to compete against each other, most women would have no chance to win, and most teams would become primarily or entirely male. Acknowledging this fact still leaves two problems, however—determining who is male and who is female, and deciding how to include transgender athletes within the male/female dichotomy.

GENDER TESTING

Medical professionals and sports organizations discussed gender testing as early as the 1930s, and because of the advantages biological males have over biological females in many popular sports, the focus was primarily on requiring those competing as women to prove that they were in fact biologically female. Interest in confirming the gender of those competing as female increased in the 1950s, with greater public awareness of male-to-female gender transition, and fears stoked by the Cold War that Communist countries might be trying to pass male athletes off as female.

Systematic gender testing was introduced at the 1966 European Athletics Championships and quickly became widespread in other competitions. These "tests" were described by those who had to undergo them as both being humiliating and based entirely on exterior appearance. Typically, a woman would be required to appear before a panel of three doctors, display their breasts and genitals to the panel, and in some cases to undergo a gynecological examination as well.

In 1967, the Barr Body test was introduced. This test was developed in the 1950s and is based on detecting the presence of a Barr body or inactive X chromosome in a somatic cell. Because women usually have one Barr Body per cell, while men have none, the presence of the Barr Body was used to determine who should be classified as biologically female. However, the Barr Body test is inaccurate for persons with non-standard chromosomes—for instance, a person with XXY chromosomes would be classified as female despite an external male appearance, and a person with X0 chromosomes would be classified as male despite an external female appearance. Despite these flaws, the Barr Body test was used by the international Olympic committee to verify gender from 1968 through 1992.

The polymerase chain reaction test, which tests for the presence of a Y chromosome (typical of males but not females) was used in the 1996 Olympics, while widespread gender testing was not employed in the 2000, 2004, or 2008 Olympics. Even in those years, however, gender testing was performed on a case-by-case basis if suspicions were raised about the gender of some female athlete. Exactly how the decision was made to test some athletes and not others is not entirely clear, but selecting people for testing based on "suspicions" raises all kinds of red flags—for instance, were women who did not present themselves in a stereotypically feminine way more likely to be selected? Were women from developing countries more likely to be selected?

The current standard for defining who is allowed to compete as female in Olympic competitions is based on the levels of natural testosterone in a person's body (the use of supplemental testosterone is a doping violation). The logic behind this rule is that men on average have higher levels of testosterone than women, and higher testosterone is considered to provide an advantage in many sports (hence many different types of illegal drugs are used to raise the testosterone level). However, as discussed in the next section, some women have naturally high levels of testosterone that overlap with the typical male range, and are higher than allowed by the Olympic standard (Caster Semenya and Dutee Chand, both discussed in the next section, are two examples). The testosterone test demonstrates once again how difficult it is to come up with a standard that can sort the variety of human beings into two discrete categories, and suggests that perhaps the effort is futile. Some argue that people should be allowed to compete in the gender category in which they live their lives, and if their bodies happen to produce high amounts of a hormone that gives them an advantage in competition, that fact should be treated no differently from the fact that some people are unusually tall or have exceptional vision, both traits that give them advantages in some sports.

TRANSGENDER AND GENDER AMBIGUOUS ATHLETES

Gender ambiguous athletes have certainly competed in sports in the past, although our knowledge is limited because systematic gender testing is a relatively recent phenomenon and because gender ambiguous people, like everyone else, are entitled to their privacy. One well-known case of a person of ambiguous gender who competed as a woman was the Polish American athlete Stella Walsh, who set many world records in athletics and won the 100 meters at the 1932 Summer Olympics. Walsh lived her entire life as a woman and only after her death in 1980 did an autopsy reveal that she had ambiguous sexual characteristics, including both XY and X0 chromosomes and an underdeveloped penis and testes. However, during Walsh's lifetime, her female gender was not questioned, while ironically one of her competitors, Helen Stephens, who won the women's 100 meters at the 1936 Summer Olympics, was forced by German officials to undergo a gender identity examination (exactly how this was conducted is unknown).

The German high jumper Dora Ratjen set a world record for the women's high jump in 1938. However, this record was disallowed when it was discovered that Ratjen had male genitals; she was issued identity papers as a man, Heinrich Ratjen, and lived the rest of his life as a man. Ratjen's story is included in the plot of the 2009 film *Berlin '36*, although the specifics of that story are disputed. In the film, Ratjen is forced to compete as a woman, in order to prevent a Jewish teammate from making the German team; a different theory proposes that Ratjen may simply have been misidentified at birth due to ambiguous genitalia and was confused about her gender identity.

Ewa Klobukowska holds the dubious distinction of being the first person to be banned from athletic competition due to a gender test. She competed in the track and field for Poland, winning a bronze medal in the 100 meters and a gold medal in the 4 100 relay at the 1964 Olympics, and breaking the world record for the 100 meters in 1965. In 1967, a chromosome test conducted before the European Cup revealed that she had mosaic XX/XXY chromosomes, and she was barred from competition. Ironically, she would have passed the Barr Body test that was used one year later at the 1968 Olympics, and even more ironically, she gave birth to a son in 1968, which would seem to many to be the ultimate proof of one's femaleness.

The Ukrainian sisters Tamara and Irina Press competed in track and field for the Soviet Union in the 1960s, setting numerous world records and winning medals in the 1960 and 1964 Olympics. Tamara won a gold medal in the shot put and a silver in the discus in 1960 and gold medals in both events in 1964, while Irina won the gold medal in the 80 meter hurdles in 1960 and in the pentathlon in 1964. Descriptions of them in the press often emphasized their "unfeminine" physiques, and they were often accused of being men, or intersex, or in some other way not "real" women. When chromosome testing was introduced in 1966, both sisters abruptly retired, and took civilian jobs within the Soviet Union.

More recently, the cases of Maria Jose Martinez-Patiño, a Spanish hurdler, Caster Semenya, a South African middle-distance runner, and Dutee Chand, an Indian sprinter, have refocused attention on the problem of determining who qualifies as female for athletic competition. Patiño, in 1986 Spain's fastest female athlete in the 100-meter hurdles, had received a physician's certificate stating that she was female, but forgot to bring it at 1986 competition, so she was required to take the Barr Body test. She failed this test, and it was discovered that her chromosomal makeup was 46, XY (typical of males), although she had the external physical appearance of a woman and had never considered herself anything but female. She was not allowed to compete as a woman and her prior victories were removed from the record books.

It was later revealed that Patiño had androgen insensitivity syndrome (AIS), a congenital condition, explaining why she had the physical external appearance of a female despite her chromosomal makeup. Patiño fought the IOC ruling and was reinstated in time to compete in the 1992 Olympics, making her the first woman to successfully challenge a gender test. However, she did not qualify for the Spanish team and thus the point became moot.

Caster Semenya, born in 1991 in South Africa, won the gold medal in the 800 meters at the World Championships in 2009. Her victory drew attention, as did her rapid improvement over the previous several years, and her physical appearance. Semenya has broad shoulders, a flat chest, narrow hips, deep voice, and an Adam's apple, which along with her athletic accomplishments raised suspicions that she was taking performance-enhancing drugs. The International Association of Athletics Federations (IAAF), the world governing body for athletics (track and field) required her to undergo gender testing; the results were not released publicly, but unofficial leaks that were covered widely in the press reported that she had intersex traits. The IAAF was sharply criticized for the way it handled the matter, with some charging that racism played a role in its insensitive treatment of Semenya.

Semenya kept a low competitive profile in 2010 and 2011, then returned to compete in the 2012 Summer Olympics, winning the silver medal in the 800 meters. Although the details of Semenya's medical history are private, many commenters noted her more feminine appearance in 2012 as well as her slower times in the 800 meters, and suggested she might be taking medication or using other means to lower her testosterone level.

Another athlete who ran afoul of gender testing rules was Dutee Chand, born in 1996 in India. She became the under-18 national champion in the 100 meters in 2012 and reached the final in the 100 meters at the 2013 World Youth Championships, becoming the first Indian to compete in the final of a world athletics event. In 2014, she was selected to compete in the Commonwealth Games, then was dropped from the team when it was discovered that she had natural levels of testosterone above that allowed by the IAAF. Chand filed a case with the Council of Arbitration for Sport (CAS), an international governing body based in Switzerland, and in 2015 CAS ruled that the IAAF testosterone rule should be suspended. While Chand has not achieved notable success at the international level, in 2016 Semenya easily won the 800 meters at the Summer Olympics, in a time faster than she ran in 2012.

Renee Richards, a tennis player, was perhaps the first transgender athlete to compete in sports at the professional level. Born Richard Raskind, Richards was a nationally ranked age-group player as a man, and after undergoing gender reassignment surgery at age 40 became a competitive female player. She sued the United States Tennis Association in 1977 when it tried to force her to take a Barr Body test before competing in the U.S. Open, arguing that the test was discriminatory under New York State law. In the 1977 case, *Renee Richards v. United States Tennis Association*, the Court ruled that a transsexual athlete should not be required to pass a gender test based on chromosomes, since such testing would not reflect the fact that they had undergone gender reassignment. The Court also gave weight to testimony by Richards's surgeon, who claimed that Richards's gender reassignment surgery reduced the level of male hormones in her body, and thus she would not have a physical advantage over cisgender women.

While Richards's success was a breakthrough for transgender people in sports, it did not fully address the question of whether a transgender woman might enjoy advantages over a cisgender woman. Some characteristics, such as height, can convey an advantage in sports and are not affected by hormone treatment or gender-affirming surgery (Richards was 6'1", considerably taller than most female players of the time). The fact that a good amateur male player could beat many of the best players in women's professional tennis, at an age when most professional players have retired, suggests that Richards enjoyed physical advantages not affected by transgender surgery (she reached the finals of the doubles championship at the U.S. Open in 1977). Richards expressed a similar thought, when reflecting on her competitive career: "I know if I'd had surgery at the age of 22, and then at 24 went on the tour, no genetic woman in the world would have been able to come close to me" (quoted in Bazelon, unpaginated).

School Sport

Some transgender athletes want to compete on high school and university sport teams, requiring administrators to deal with issues they may not have previously considered. In 2009, a "national think tank" was convened including leaders from the National Collegiate Athletic Association (NCAA) and the National High School Federation, as well as experts from the fields of law, medicine, athletics, and advocacy, and transgender student athletes. In 2010, the participants in this endeavor released a report, "On the Team: Equal Opportunity for Transgender Student Athletes," which includes a number of recommendations for policies regarding transgender student athletes.

"On the Team" begins by noting that inclusion and equal opportunity in education are core values, and that basic issues of fairness and equity should include all students. Legal decisions in many regions have also added gender identity as a protected category, so that discrimination against transgender people is a violation of the law. No one knows how many transgender students there are in the United States, but the number appears to be increasing, so it is vital that schools have policies in place to meet their needs. At the same time, adult leadership can provide models of tolerance for cisgender students, and learning about transgender students can help everyone understand issues of sex and gender more completely.

School sports programs have long been treated in the United States as fundamental to the educational enterprise, both for the opportunities they offer for students to learn and compete in sports, and also for inculcating values such as fair play, teamwork, and the rewards of focused working toward a goal. Regulations regarding transgender students should take into account the age of the student and medical recommendations regarding the treatment of transgender students.

For instance, for children in grade school, it may be appropriate for them to assume their chosen gender identity in terms of dress and social function, but without medical intervention. For children approaching puberty, hormone blockers may be appropriate to prevent the development of secondary sex characteristics that conflict with their core identity. For older high school and college students, hormone treatment or surgery may be appropriate.

One reason the participation of transgender athletes is concerning to some students and adults is that the transgender individual may enjoy a competitive advantage, particularly when transgender individuals assigned male gender at birth compete on the same teams as cisgender girls. This is more of a concern after athletes reach puberty, particularly if the transgender athlete is not using blocking hormones to delay the onset of secondary sexual characteristics. In such cases, it is worth remembering that transgender students are relatively rare, and that transgender students often face discrimination and harassment, making it unlikely that anyone would pretend to be transgender simply for the opportunity to compete on a girls' team. It is also worth remembering that both males and females exist in a range of body sizes and types, and so even a boy who has begun puberty will not necessarily enjoy a large advantage over most girls.

According to the best available medical evidence, most athletic advantages due to gender are gone after a year of hormone treatment (except for permanent changes, such as the size and shape of the skeleton, which have not been studied), so transgender and cisgender females can compete on a fairly equal basis. Given the importance of gender identity in a person's functioning, it must be considered if that possibility of advantage outweighs the many benefits of allowing transgender students to compete in the gender of their choice.

POLICY RECOMMENDATIONS

"On the Team," the 2010 report written by Pat Griffin and Helen J. Carroll produced in conjunction with the National Center for Lesbian Rights, the Women's Sports Foundation, and It Takes a Team! includes series of recommendations for inclusion of transgender student athletes in high school and college sports. These are based on the way sport is organized in the United States but may be applicable in general principle to other countries as well. These recommendations are founded on a series of ten guiding principles:

1. Participation in interscholastic and intercollegiate athletics is a valuable part of the education experience for all students.
2. Transgender student athletes should have equal opportunity to participate in sports.
3. The integrity of women's sports should be preserved.
4. Policies governing sports should be based on sound medical knowledge and scientific validity.
5. Policies governing sports should be objective, workable, and practicable, and should also be written, available, and equitably enforced.
6. Policies governing the participation of transgender students should be fair in light of the tremendous variation among individuals in strength, size, musculature, and ability.
7. The legitimate privacy interests of all student athletes should be protected.
8. The medical privacy of transgender students should be preserved.
9. Athletic administrators, staff, parents of athletes, and student athletes should have access to sound and effective educational resources and training related to the participation of transgender and gender-variant students in athletics.
10. Policies governing the participation of transgender students in athletes should comply with state and federal laws protecting students from discrimination based on sex, disability, and gender identity and expression. (Griffin and Carroll, "On the Team," 21–22)

For high school athletics, "On the Team" recommends that athletes be allowed to participate in sports based on their gender identity, whether or not it conflicts with the gender identity listed on their birth certificate, and without any requirement that they have undertaken medical treatment based on their gender identity. The document also spells out a recommended process for notifying school and state officials that an athlete has a gender identity different from that listed on his or her birth certificate. It also prescribes an appeal process with standards for documentation should there be questions about a student's gender identity or eligibility to participate in sport.

For college athletes, "On the Team" recommends that transgender athletes be allowed to participate, with specific rules governing the use of hormone treatment. Basically, a male-to female athlete may participate on a woman's team after one year of hormone treatment and can participate on a men's team at any time. A female-to-male athlete cannot compete on a woman's team after beginning hormone treatment and must apply for an exemption to compete on a men's team (because taking testosterone supplements is generally prohibited but can be allowed for transgender transition). In any case, the hormone treatment must be monitored by a physician.

For transgender athletes not taking hormones related to gender transition, the student may participate in sports based on gender as assigned at birth. Female-to male transgender athletes not taking hormones may participate on a men's team, but male-to-female transgender athletes may not participate on a women's team. In mixed gender teams, a female-to-male transgender athlete not taking hormone treatments may be counted as either male or female, while male-to-female transgender athletes not taking hormone treatments will count as a man.

"On the Team" also includes guidelines on other aspects of transgender athlete inclusion. Transgender athletes should be allowed to use facilities such as locker rooms based on their gender identity and be assigned roommates based on their gender identity. The transgender athlete should be referred to using their chosen names and preferred pronouns. Uniforms should be appropriate to the sport and the individual's gender identity, and regulations regarding off-the-field clothing (e.g., dress codes during team travel) should be gender-neutral. Everyone involved in sport, including media, should be educated about the needs of transgender athletes, but without violating the confidentiality of any particular athlete. Athletic departments should discipline individuals who violate policies regarding transgender athletes (e.g., by breaching confidentiality), and retaliation should be forbidden against anyone who complains about discrimination based on gender identity or expression.

ALTERNATIVES TO THE BINARY GENDER MODELS

Most competitive sport at the elite level, and often at the non-elite, is organized assuming that there are only two genders, male and female, and that participants will fit neatly into one category or the other. The need to find some way to include transgender athletes in sport, while also being fair to cisgender males and females, has led some to propose alternative ways to organize sport.

Adam Love proposes that sporting officials and scholars abandon the sex-binary-based model for organizing sports competitions and instead embrace a broader and more inclusive model. He assumes that sex and gender are categories constructed socially and historically rather than biological absolutes (his analysis concerns transgender rather than intersex athletes, i.e., those whose sexual identification is different from their sex assigned at birth, rather than those with characteristics of both sexes).

Love points to the fact that concerns about determining the gender of competitive athletes may be based not only on concerns about fairness but also about social expectations concerning what is appropriate for men and women. Muscles and strength are commonly associated in Western societies with men, for instance, and women who present "too much" of these characteristics may be felt to threaten this assumption. Hormonal testing was one attempt to answer this concern, but the variety of hormonal patterns present in human beings demonstrated that this approach was not sufficient. Other attempts to impose the male/female dichotomy, through rules based on anatomy or hormones, has had the paradoxical effect of demonstrating that many individuals do not fit the neat categories of "opposite" sexes. Love also points out that while gender testing has resulted in the ban of some intersex athletes, it has turned up no cases of deliberate gender fraud.

As an alternative to binary-sex-based leagues, Love points to some lesbian softball leagues in the United States that specifically include transgender men and women as well as those whose gender identity may not fit gender binary categories. He points to the ability of such leagues to act as sites of support for transgender individuals, and the possibility that interactions between transgender and cisgender athletes will lessen prejudices. He also points that such inclusion may help to challenge orthodox notions of masculinity and femininity in sports as a whole.

Love decries rules regarding transgender athletes that assume women are biologically inferior in terms of sports but fails to address the reality that in many popular sports that is unambiguously the case. While it is not true that every male athlete is superior in every way to every female athlete, it is also true that at high levels of competition, the best male athletes are far superior to the best female athletes. While this distinction may not be important in recreational sports leagues, it is crucial for ensuring fair competition at the elite level. Were men and women forced to compete against each other in popular sports such as athletics or basketball, men would dominate the competitions and most women would never be in the running.

CHAPTER 9

Normative Gender Dichotomies and Alternatives

To many people, there's no mystery about gender—there are only two possibilities, male or female, the categories are distinct, and everyone fits neatly into one or the other. This dichotomous way of conceptualizing gender is common and, for many people, adequate. However, for some people, the question of gender is more complex, and they find the dichotomous, fixed model of gender inadequate to describe themselves. This chapter looks at the motives for classifying people by gender, some consequences of the dichotomous system, and attempts to create alternative ways of describing gender. It also looks at gender policing and how it affects both cisgender and transgender people.

WHY CLASSIFY PEOPLE BY GENDER CATEGORIES?

One may begin by asking what purpose is served by classifying people into a fixed number of gender categories. Certainly various systems have been developed over the years, and the dichotomous male/female model is only one possibility among several. But a more fundamental question is why anyone would feel the need to develop a theory that specifies a specific number of gender categories and classifies people into one category. This sentiment is summed up in a phrase attributed to Mickey Diamond, a professor at the University of Hawaii School of Medicine: "Nature loves variety. Unfortunately, society hates it" (in Amy Bloom, *Normal: Transsexual CEOs, Crossdressing Cops, and Hermaphrodites with Attitude.* New York: Vintage, 2003, p. 135).

One answer is that part of the work of scientists is to observe and classify nature, and that often such efforts are not only benign but actually useful. Chemistry would not have advanced far without the work of the many scientists who identified the different elements and their characteristics, for instance, and the periodic table of the elements is an essential tool used by scientists and science students alike. The development of taxonomies to classify plants and animals is another example of a system of classification that has helped increase our understanding of the complex world around us as well as providing structure for scientific work.

However, it is also useful to bear in mind is that no system of classification, however useful, is necessarily the final word on the subject. Instead, like all scientific theories, systems of classification are open to revision as scientific knowledge increases. In the 18th century, the Swedish scientist Carl Linnaeus created the modern system of taxonomy used to classify organisms. This was an important scientific breakthrough, and scientists today are still using a version of the system created by Linnaeus to classify new organisms. However, the taxonomy as developed by Linnaeus has been revised many times to incorporate new knowledge, some of which was achieved through the use of technology not available in Linnaeus's day, such as high-powered microscopes. For instance, Linnaeus based his system on the physical appearance of organisms and at the highest level of classification included just two kingdoms, *Plantae* (plants) and *Animalia* (animals). Today, scientists are more interested in classifying organisms based on their common ancestry and have proposed systems of classification including as many as seven kingdoms. Other scientists argue that the category of kingdom is no longer useful and should be abandoned. Such disagreements and revisions are a normal part of science—ideas are always open to examination and revision as our knowledge of the world increases and as new theories are developed and tested to explain different aspects of it.

Another point is that while developing systems to classify the world around us is a normal product of human curiosity, and has often proved scientifically useful, sorting simple organisms into categories is quite a different enterprise from imposing fixed categories on human beings. Another distinction is that taxonomic categories are meant to describe relationships among organisms, rather than as a means to prescribe how they should behave. To take an absurd example, the phylogenetic system of classification recognizes that birds are related to reptiles, but no one would take that information as a directive to try to make birds to become more like reptiles, let alone force them into conversion therapy! And yet the fact that many people endorse the classification of people into exactly two genders, with specific characteristics and behaviors prescribed for each, has resulted in efforts to make nonconforming people fit the classification system (from gender-conforming surgery performed on infants to so-called conversion therapy that attempts to make gay people into heterosexuals) rather than revising the system to fit the variety of human existence, or discarding the binary system of gender categories altogether.

LEARNING WHAT IT MEANS TO BE MALE OR FEMALE

Learning what it means to be male or female in a particular society is a complex process, and one that begins at a surprisingly early age. Various studies, summarized by Anne Fausto-Sterling in *Sex/Gender*, show that adults interact differently with infants based on the infant's assumed gender beginning in the first months of life, and such differences are more subtle than simply calling a girl baby beautiful and charming and a boy baby strong and handsome. For instance, mothers are more likely to interact with girls face to face, while they are more likely to interact physically with boys. Children as young as three or four months old can tell the difference between male and female voices and seem to differentiate between male and female faces as well. By about one year, children can associate male or female voices with faces of the appropriate gender.

By their second year, children have learned to associate some objects, such as hammers, fire hats, and bears, with males, and by the third year children begin to express their gender identity and can describe themselves as either a boy or a girl; the concept that gender is a fixed property seems to emerge later, around age seven. So children learn long before they are ready to attend school that certain behaviors and activities are coded as male, others as female, and that a behavior such as a man putting on lipstick is a violation of those norms. However, these developments are partly cultural in nature (what is considered appropriate for boys versus girls, or men versus women, differs from one society to the next) and is also influenced by the makeup of one's family. For instance, three-year-olds who have an older sibling of the same sex—a boy with an older brother, or a girl with an older sister—have been shown to display more behaviors associated with their sex, and fewer of those associated with the opposite sex. In contrast, children with more educated parents have been shown to adhere less strictly to behaviors societally coded as appropriate for their sex, as compared to children of less educated parents.

Although most children identify themselves as the gender they were assigned at birth, a subset does not. Children as young as three may identify themselves as belonging to the opposite gender, but such children are not necessarily homogeneous in their reasons for claiming an identity other than the one applied to them at birth. In other words, we can observe that some children feel their true gender is not the one assigned them at birth, but we don't yet know the reasons that motivate them to make that declaration. This aspect of gender identity in childhood is not yet well understood, but what is known is that not all children who persistently identify as the opposite gender at a young age maintain that identity through adolescence and adulthood. For instance, Fausto-Sterling cites a study from the Netherlands that identifies two groups among adolescents who sought treatment from a Gender Identity Clinic when they were seven to ten years old: "persisters" who continued to have gender dysphoria in adolescence, and "desisters" who came to be comfortable with the bodies they were born with and with gender-conforming activities. The fact that not all children who identify as transgender continue to do so in adolescence, however, does not suggest that their earlier self-identification was invalid, but simply that gender identity is complex and there is much we do not yet know about it.

CONSEQUENCES OF THE NORMATIVE GENDER DICHOTOMY

One obvious consequence of the belief in the normative gender dichotomy is that people who did not fit into either category neatly may be ostracized, or worse. Boys who are perceived as effeminate, for instance, may be taunted and bullied, as may girls whose appearance or behavior is judged to be "too masculine." For transgender individuals, this problem is even worse, as they may find total strangers demanding that they explain themselves and their gender, with a type of invasive questioning that would not be applied to someone who presented a standard cisgender appearance. Transgender individuals may also choose to deny their trans identity because it causes them so many problems in daily life and try to fulfill the stereotypes of whichever gender they find the easiest fit. It's not entirely clear why so many people should be so insistent on defending the standard male/female dichotomy, other than the fact that it seems natural to them, and that many cultural habits are based on the belief that there are only two genders.

The broad acceptance of two gender categories and related beliefs about the characteristics of men and women has broad consequences for individuals who fit into this schema, as well as for those who do not. Many social customs depend on knowing whether a person is male or female, from forms of address (do you call an adult as "sir" or "ma'am"?) to courtesies (who holds the door for whom, who gets out of the elevator first?). Many people may feel uncomfortable if they don't recognize someone as obviously male or female, in part because they have learned different expectations to apply to each gender. Dress codes for schools and workplaces are typically based on the conventional male/female dichotomy, and most public restrooms are still classified as being for either men or women.

Classifying people as male or female is something everyone does on a regular basis, and with that classification comes a variety of beliefs about men and women that may be unconscious but may still guide the believer's actions. Such decisions may be made in person, but also remotely, for instance, based on an individual's name or the sound of their voice. These unstated beliefs have been proposed as one factor in the wage gap between men and women, which has persisted in many countries, despite laws explicitly banning discrimination on the basis of gender. For instance, a study by Corinne Moss-Racusin found that when science faculty were sent fictional resumes identical in every way except for the name of the "applicant," the "applicants" with male names were judged as more competent, were more likely to be offered a job, and were offered a higher salary, than were the "applicants" with female names. Similarly, an experiment designed by Lillian MacNell, Adam Driscoll, and Andrea N. Hunt found that students in an online course gave higher teacher evaluations to instructors they believed were male and lower evaluations to instructors they believed were female, independent of the actual gender of the person teaching the course (the students never met their teacher, so they judged the teacher's gender based on their name).

Even in less obvious ways, people's beliefs about men and women can lead to biased conclusions. For instance, many people believe women talk more than men, and stereotypes such as the talkative gossip are typically applied only to women. A study by Anne Cutler and Donia R. Scott investigated whether this belief might be due not to the fact that women talk more than men, but that in a given conversation people typically overestimate the amount of talking done by women and underestimate the amount done by men. In their study, they had people listen to taped conversations in which men and women spoke exactly the same number of words, and found that in mixed-gender conversations, listeners believed that women had spoken more. This misperception has real-life implications—for instance, women may learn to speak less in order to not appear pushy or domineering—and also underlines the fact that even in very basic matters when gender should not matter at all, it is common to make assumptions based on the perceived gender of individuals.

ALTERNATIVES TO THE MALE/FEMALE DICHOTOMY

Even if one believes that humans can be classified into a specific number of genders, that number does not necessarily have to be two. In fact, while the male/female dichotomy has been commonly accepted for centuries, and those who fall outside (e.g., people with physical characteristics of both genders) frequently condemned as defective, this dichotomy has also been challenged by various other systems. In the 19th century, the German writer and activist Karl Heinrich Ulrichs published a number of papers in which he developed what became known as "third sex theory" to explain homosexuality. Ulrichs used the term *Urning* to describe someone who was born with a male body but had a "female soul" and was attracted to other men, while the feminine version of this word, *Urningin*, was used to describe someone born with a female body but who had a "male soul" and was attracted to other women. He also used the term *Zwitter* to describe an intersex or transgender person. A similar term, *Uranian*, was used by English writers in the 19th century to refer to male homosexuals.

The German physician and sex researcher Magnus Hirschfeld, who conducted groundbreaking research into sexual minorities and was also a political activist who tried to overturn legislation outlawing homosexual behavior, developed a theory of gender and sexuality that allowed for a continuum of types, rather than a strict number of discrete categories. This theory used the German term *Zwischenstufen* (intermediate steps or intermediate types) to express the concept that many different variants of gender and sexuality exist in nature and should be considered normal.

More recently, the American biologist Anne Fausto-Sterling has suggested five gender categories: male, female, true hermaphrodites or herms (individuals who possess one testes and one ovary), male hermaphrodites or merms (individuals with testes and some female genitalia, but no ovaries), and female hermaphrodites or merms who have ovaries and some male genitalia but no testes. Fausto-Sterling is not entirely serious in offering these categories for consideration, however—her real point is that any discrete number of categories will not be sufficient to describe the variety of gender and sexuality among human beings. Other systems to classify individuals by sex or gender have also been developed over the years, and more will undoubtedly be developed in the future, but it's always worth remembering that the reality of human diversity is one thing and attempts to describe that diversity with a set number of categories is just that—an attempt to impose man-made categories on nature's infinite variety.

Interestingly, some young people today seem to be rejecting the dichotomous system of gender classification. For instance, a January 2015 telephone poll conducted by the Benenson Strategy Group, based on a national sample of 1,000 people aged 18 through 34, found that less than half (46%) endorsed the view that there are only two genders, male and female, while 50 percent endorsed the concept of a gender spectrum with some people falling outside the conventional categories. The same poll found differences in opinion by several demographic categories as well. Support was strongest for the gender spectrum concept among those aged 18–24 (57%) and weakest among those aged 30–34 (49%). Women (57%) were more likely than men (44%) to endorse the concept of a gender spectrum, as were people who described their ideology as liberal (75%) rather than moderate (52%) or conservative (30%). Support for the gender spectrum was highest among those with a college education (54%), as opposed to those who had only attended high school (43%), and was highest in the Northeast region (58%) and lowest in the South (42%).

GENDER POLICING

As noted earlier, there is widespread if sometimes unconscious acceptance of the belief that there are exactly two genders, male and female, and every person fits neatly into one or the other. For many people, the presence of an individual who does not fit this rigid dichotomy may induce feeling ranging from confusion to fear to panic, because the very existence of that individual challenges assumptions so basic that they may be unconscious. These responses to a person who does not fit the assumed categories can give rise to gender policing, in which someone takes upon themselves, unasked, the job of imposing gender categories on other people. As the name "policing" suggests, individuals who take part in gender policing often act as if it were their job to evaluate other people's appearance and behavior against some checklist of gender appropriateness, without considering that other people may be operating from entirely different points of view.

While the term *gender policing* may be unfamiliar to many people, the concept certainly is not. When someone mocks a man for wearing pink because it is a "girls' color," or a woman is rebuked for speaking her mind because she's "acting like a man," those are examples of gender policing, because someone is trying to impose a set of gender-based rules and categories on individuals who may be operating from an entirely different set of standards. Gender policing attempts to restrict the choices of people by imposing penalties, from simple social disapproval to the threat of violence or legal prosecution, on choices that do not conform with the rules and categories in the mind of a person who believes they have the right to make such judgments. In fact, gender policing is so common that it may not be perceived as such—instead, it may simply seem like a normal part of the social fabric.

Gender policing can affect anyone, including cisgender men and women. For instance, a cisgender woman who chooses to not wear makeup, high heels, or dresses may be criticized for not being feminine enough or accused of being a lesbian, when in fact she is simply dressing in a way that is comfortable and feels normal to her. Even if she performs well in her job and is always well-groomed, she may be passed over for promotions at work due to her nonconformist personal presentation. If she speaks up in meetings without first engaging in a series of self-deprecations, she may be judged as "pushy" or "overbearing," even if her manner of speaking is not different from the men in her company. A female teacher may be expected to take on emotional labor (e.g., helping students with personal problems), while no such expectation is placed on male teachers, and if the female teacher declines this additional burden she may be criticized while the men simply are never asked to perform this labor. Similarly, a man may be criticized for wearing clothing that is judged not sufficiently masculine by someone's arbitrary and unstated standards, or for declining to engage in locker room talk, and those judgments may hurt his career even if his job performance is excellent.

Although gender policing restricts everyone's choices, transgender people are even more likely to be affected by it than cisgender people, and the consequences are far more likely to be severe. Both transgender children and adults have been bullied, attacked, and even killed because someone decided that their presentation or behavior did not fit some arbitrary gender schema. In addition, some cities still have laws on the books that make it a crime to appear in public as a gender other than the one to which you were assigned at birth. The passage of "bathroom bills" that make it a crime to use a public restroom based on your gender identity rather than your gender as assigned at birth encourages gender policing, by suggesting that it is the duty of private citizens to take on the task of evaluating the gender of anyone using a public restroom. Such bathroom bills are often justified by appealing to an unfounded but apparently widely believed belief that women are likely to be attacked, in public restrooms by men masquerading as women. They also appeal to a certain conformist mind-set, by providing a way for women whose outward appearance is not traditionally feminine to be singled out and embarrassed in public.

CHAPTER 10

Parenting and Family Issues

Most people have experienced being part of a family, but what constitutes a family is defined culturally and historically. For instance, at one time in the United States, the standard definition of a family assumed it to consist of two married parents and their dependent biological children (a so-called nuclear family). Of course, many families have never fit that definition, and today we recognize that a much broader range of social groups can constitute a family. While the specific functions of a family may vary from one context to another, common functions of a family include providing social, economic, and emotional support for family members. Not all families include parents and children, but many do, including families in which one or more of the members are transgender. Transgender parents, and the parents of transgender children, face many challenges in common with all parents, as well as some issues relating to the transgender status of the parent and/or child, and the discrimination and misunderstanding sometimes faced by transgender people in our society.

TYPES OF PARENTING

There are many ways that a trans person can be a parent, just as there are many ways for cisgender people to be parents. Biological parents are usually defined as the man and woman who contributed genetic material (sperm and ovum) to the fertilized egg that became the child, and may or may not be the same people who raise the child.

One common type of parenting that does not fit this exact definition is the practice of helping raise a partner's children. In the past, this relationship was typically referred to with the prefix "step" (i.e., stepmother, stepfather) but that practice has become less common as blended families have become more common. Trans people face the same issues as cisgender people with this type of parenting (e.g., will the child accept you as a parent?) as well as trans-specific issues. For instance, other family members may not accept the trans parent as a "real" parent, and if the partner is in a custody battle, the former partner may use the new partner's trans status to argue in court that the household is unsuitable for rearing children. The trans parent will also have to decide when and how to discuss his or her trans status with the partner's children.

Some trans people choose to adopt children or to serve as foster parents. All people applying to be adoptive or foster parents must go through a rigorous vetting process (understandably, for the protection of the children who may be placed in the household), but the mere fact of an individual's trans status should not be held against them. Some states have laws banning same-sex adoption, but no state has a law against a transgender person adopting or serving as a foster parent. In reality, however, such decisions are made by human beings who may hold prejudices about such matters, and bias on the part of a judge or other official may mean that an otherwise qualified adoptive or foster parent is discriminated against. Suggestions from *Trans Bodies, Trans Selves* to improve the probability of a successful adoption or fostering include working with an agency looking for trans foster parents, working with agencies that are comfortable with gay and lesbian prospective parents, letting the agency know early in the process that you are trans, retaining an attorney familiar with trans issues and adoptions or foster care, and consulting with a therapist who would be willing to testify to your fitness as a parent.

Some trans people are biological parents. Those planning to transition who want to preserve the option of being biological parents should consider the probable effects of the transition process on their fertility and plan accordingly. If removal of the testicles or ovaries is planned, it is possible to preserve sperm and eggs or fertilized ova cryogenically (cisgender people also do this, e.g., if they must have cancer treatments that will make them sterile). The effects of hormone treatment on fertility are less certain, but some reports indicate that irreversible sterility may result after as little as three months of treatment. On the other hand, some trans men have successfully become pregnant and given birth despite years of taking testosterone.

It's also possible to become a parent through the use of donated or purchased sperm and/or eggs, and it is also possible to use a surrogate to carry the pregnancy to term and give birth to the baby. Techniques like artificial insemination and in vitro fertilization (IVF) are available to transgender people, as they are to cisgender people.

TRANSGENDER PEOPLE AS PARENTS

The choice to become a parent is highly personal and individual. As with cisgender people, not all transgender people desire to be parents, but many do. Until recently, little information was available about transgender parenting, and many people might have considered the very concept absurd. This is a mistaken attitude that can be corrected through education. In fact, many transgender people are parents today, and many more will become parents in the future.

Parenting is a big job, and transgender people may worry that they are not up to the task (many cisgender people share the same worry!). They may also worry about a lack of social support for themselves and their children, particularly if they are estranged from their own families. Finally, they may be worried that something about their transgender status may preclude their being good parents, although that worry is clearly misplaced based on the available research.

Rebecca Stotzer and colleagues published a review of the scientific literature on transgender parenting, including the results of 51 studies. They found that although transgender people are parents at a lower rate than the general population, a substantial number of transgender people are parents; one study estimated that 700,000 transgender adults in the United States are parents, while the percentage of transgender people who are parents ranged from 15.0 percent to 46.2 percent, depending on the study. By way of comparison, about two-thirds of American adults report being parents. While different studies found different rates of parenting, in general transgender women are more likely than transgender men to report that they are parents, while a comparison of rates of parenting among gender nonconforming individuals shows a wide range across different studies. Parenting rates also seem to be higher among those whose transition or "come out" as transgender occurred later in life, perhaps because those individuals became parents while they were living in the gender to which they were assigned at birth. Although only a few studies had sufficient transgender parent respondents to allow a breakdown by race and ethnicity, one study found the highest rate of both being a parent and having a dependent child among American Indians, with the lowest rates among Asians, and the rates for Hispanics, blacks, whites, and multiracial individuals falling between those two groups.

Transgender people are often discriminated against as parents, and may find their transgender status used against them at custody hearings. While there are no laws specifically barring transgender people from adopting or fostering children, there are also few laws to protect their rights as adoptive or foster parents. Transgender people may also face child custody and/ or visitation challenges when a relationship ends, as some have found that their trans status alone may be assumed by the court system to be evidence of their unfitness as a parent. Despite this discrimination, many transgender people report living with children (the rate ranged from 2.5 percent to 33.3 percent, depending on the study).

Parenting is a difficult job, and all parents need support. Several studies have looked specifically at the needs of transgender parents and found that they deal with issues similar to those of cisgender parents, with top issues including access to child care, need for parenting skills training, the desire to network with other parents, the need for support groups that could address their issues, and the need for family planning services. Some also cited the need for more information and support for transgender parents during the transition process, and some have reported difficulty in obtaining support and assistance even from organizations founded to help gay and bisexual parents.

Child Well-Being

Most transgender parents report having positive relationships with their children; for instance, the 2004 Idaho Tobacco Prevention and Control Program found that 78.9 percent of transgender parents said their relationship with their child or children was positive or very positive, and 73.7 percent said their experience of raising their child or children was overall positive or very positive; both rates are similar to those reported by non-transgender parents in the same study. A separate study by Stephen Erich and colleagues in 2008 found that 60.5 percent of transgender people with children reported having a good or excellent relationship with their children.

Transgender parents may worry about the effect of their transition on their children. The results may be varied, according to information drawn from the National Transgender Discrimination Study, which found that 22 percent of respondents reported the child-parent relationship improved after the parent's transition, 36 percent reported that it remained about the same, 13 percent reported that some things got better while others got worse, and 29 percent said the relationship was worse following transition. Other studies have found that most transgender parents report mostly positive or no change in their relationship with their children following transition, although a minority does report that the relationship worsened. Several studies have identified factors that are associated with positive adjustment by a child to a parent's transition, including the child having close emotional ties to the non-transitioning parent, parental cooperation in child-rearing, support of the extended family for the transitioning parent, the child having a close relationship with the transitioning parent, and the child having ongoing contact with both parents. Some studies have also found that it is easier for young children to adapt to having a transgender parent than older or young adult children.

Only a few studies have been conducted evaluating the well-being of children with transgender parents, and some of the available studies were conducted with small samples. Nonetheless, the available evidence suggests that there is no harm to a child in having a transgender parent, nor does there seem to be any impact on the child's gender identity or sexual orientation. While some children may suffer teasing or harassment from their peers due to their having a transgender parent, this appears to be relatively limited.

Trans-Specific Issues in Parenting

There are some specific issues that trans parents must deal with. One is deciding at what age children should learn of the parent's transgender status, and in what detail this needs to be discussed; both are individual issues that depend on the maturity of the child, among other things. Parents should remember that children have their own minds and concerns, and it may be natural for them to reject the parent's new status for a while, or to mourn a parent they believe they are losing.

Trans Bodies, Trans Selves suggests some questions that trans parents may want to ask themselves before discussing their trans status with their children. These include whether the parent will be changing his or her name, and what name they want the child to call them; whether the transition will include hormones or surgery, and what kind of changes that may bring; what the parent wants the children to tell their friends, teachers, and friends' parents about the transition, if anything; whether parental personality changes should be expected during the transition; what role the parent will play after the transition (father, mother, or something else?) and how they want the child to address them.

PARENTING A TRANSGENDER CHILD

It's an almost mythical scene—a baby is born, and the first words out of the delivering doctor's or midwife's mouth are "It's a boy!" or "It's a girl!" Today, of course, many parents know the apparent gender of their child before birth, thanks to ultrasound. Advances in scientific technology hasn't changed the fact that in many people's minds, a baby is either a boy or a girl, based on the appearance of the external genitals, and that is that. For many people, it really is that simple—their external genitals, their internal sense of gender, their chromosomes, and every other method of defining gender are in alignment. However, for some fraction of individuals, their experience is at odds with the gender assigned at birth. While less than 1 percent of the population may experience this discrepancy, that's still a substantial number of people, and of course to those people the issue is very real indeed.

Although it may seem strange to be concerned about the gender of preschool children or even children in primary school, our society makes many assumptions about how children should dress and behave based on gender. When I was in grade school, every time we left the classroom (e.g., to go to recess), we formed one line of boys and another of girls, and of course the school restrooms were segregated by gender. Failing to fit into one category or the other may result in many awkward situations, so parents may find it difficult to let a child be gender nonconforming outside the home, and yet their child may be very unhappy in the gender they were assigned at birth.

There is no absolute definition or checklist to determine who is transgender and who is not. Instead, physicians and others trained to work with transgender children look at patterns of behavior and clusters, and parents are advised to seek out assistance from someone familiar with transgender issues. Many children display some gender nonconforming behavior (e.g., a girl may prefer to play with trucks than dolls), but this does not necessarily indicate that the child is transgender. However, some children also repeatedly and over a period of time make statements like "I'm not a girl, I'm a boy!" and "Why do you keep saying 'she' when I'm a 'he'?" If such behavior persists, and if the child seems to be very unhappy when pressed to do something associated with their birth gender (e.g., wearing a bathing suit appropriate to his or her birth gender), parents may want to seek out professional assistance. One standard used in psychiatry is that gender dysphoria in childhood requires a child to experience a period of at least six months in which they feel a difference between their gender as assigned at birth and their experienced gender, and that they must feel distress or impairment as a result.

Children's sense of gender identity may shift over time, and it's worth remembering that children have a limited understanding of sex roles and a limited vocabulary to discuss their feelings and experiences. Sometimes behaviors and declarations that seem to adults to be indicative of transgender identity may just be instances of gender nonconformity: children can observe that there are boys and girls, and that certain behaviors, clothing, and attitudes are associated with each, while they are unlikely to be familiar with terms like *genderqueer* or the concepts behind them.

It is important for parents to accept their child's sense of gender as it is, and to be supportive, because a transgender child will undoubtedly face misunderstanding and opposition in the outside world. Parents also need to recognize and process their own emotions, as even the most understanding parents may not be familiar with the reality of raising a transgender child. They may feel like the child's identity places an extra burden on them, and in some sense they are right—life is harder when you don't fit the societally defined categories of male and female, and in the case of dependent children parents will have more battles than usual to fight for their child. Parents may also grieve the loss of the child they thought they had, deny or fear the child's transgender status, or feel guilty ("What did we do wrong?") that their child is not "normal." These are normal emotions, and one of the best things parents can do for their children is to educate themselves and seek whatever counseling they need so they can assist the child on his or her journey through life. Besides professional counseling, there are support groups for children of transgender children (if no one can provide you with a referral, you can find such groups by searching the Internet). There are also many recent books and films about transgender children and their families that may help provide parents with guidance as well as making them feel less alone.

Social Transition

Young children and their parents may decide that the child should go through a social transition in which they will express their gender identity in public. This may include making changes in the child's name, in pronouns used to refer to the child, and in the child's appearance (hairstyle, clothing, etc.) and behavior (e.g., preferred toys). This "coming out" may be planned as a gradual process, with the child revealing his or her preferred identity to a small group of trusted relatives and friends, then extending it to school (with suitable preparations with the teachers beforehand), and eventually the chosen identity becoming the child's new norm.

Not everyone is familiar with transgender issues, and not everyone is welcoming of difference (in gender as in other matters), so children should be prepared for negative reactions. Parent should anticipate the kinds of questions that the child may be asked, and practice role playing so the

3

child is comfortable making appropriate responses (and recognizing when a question is inappropriate and need not be answered). A similar approach can be taken if the child wishes to select a new name—parents and child can work together to select something all parties feel is appropriate, and practice using it at home and then with a selected group of friends.

If the child is old enough to attend school, it's important that they be able to use their preferred gender identity there. The burden of making this happen falls primarily on the child's parents, who need to inform school teachers and administrators of the situation. While many schools are eager to be inclusive and help transgender children fit into the life of the school, others are unaware of best practices in this regard. Parents can help by informing the school of model policies in school systems, such as the Seattle Public Schools, that have been leaders in addressing the needs of transgender children. Parents also need to be aware that their transgender child may become the target of bullies and to be proactive in addressing this issue. If the child has been attending school using their birth gender identity, parents may consider moving them to another school for a "fresh start" with students and staff who didn't know their previous identity, but this is a choice to be considered rather than a universal rule.

Medical Interventions

As a transgender child approaches puberty, parents will want to consult with medical professionals on the options available to their child. Individuals assigned female at birth typically begin puberty between 9 and 11 years old (the first signs typically include the emergence of breast buds and sometimes a small amount of pubic hair), while those assigned male at birth typically begin puberty between ages 11 and 13 (the first signs are typically increased testicular volume and possibly a small amount of pubic hair). It is possible to use drugs known as "puberty blockers" (most commonly analogs of gonadotropin-releasing hormone or GnRH) to delay the onset of puberty and allow the child and parent more time to make decisions about the child's gender. Delaying the decision until a child is 16 or 17 means that their body will go through the changes of puberty, most of which are permanent or semipermanent and can only be changed later through surgery, if at all. Some changes that take place during puberty, such as the differing skeletal characteristics and facial structure of adult men and women, are very difficult to disguise or change. In contrast, the effects of puberty blockers are reversible, so that if the child decides to stop taking the medication, the changes of puberty will occur as they would have without the interruption.

Some adolescents may also want to take cross-sex hormones—estrogen for trans girls and testosterone for trans boys. These drugs will aid in the development of physical characteristics associated with their gender identity, such as, for trans females, development of breast tissue, softer skin, and redistribution of body fat, and for trans males, development of a deep voice, growth of body and facial hair, growth of the clitoris, fat redistribution, and cessation of menstrual periods. These changes may be permanent or semipermanent, and thus the decision to begin cross-sex hormones should be considered carefully. Cross-sex hormones may result in sterility after only a few months of treatment, so this fact should also be considered before treatment is begun.

One consideration in administering cross-sex hormones is that they may allow a child to mature into his or her chosen gender identity at the same rate as his or her peer group. This desire must be balanced, of course, against the fact that the effects of cross-sex hormones may not be reversible. Girls go through puberty several years earlier than boys, so if it is a goal to keep a trans girl "in sync" with her peer group in terms of sexual development, this should be kept in mind.

CHAPTER 11

Research Issues

Any social science researcher must deal with methodological issues, but the study of transgender people poses particular challenges that complicate the research process and also make it difficult to compare results from different studies. First is the difficulty in finding people willing to participate in research—because transgender people are often the focus of discrimination and harassment, they may be reluctant to come forward, and to be open about sharing aspects of their lives, particularly with a researcher they may perceive as an outsider wanting to exploit them. Another problem is the lack of common definition of what it means to be transgender, a problem common to studying sexuality in general—should the definition of one's sex or gender be based on personal identification, societal identification, behavior, or some combination of those factors alone with others? Additional complications arise from the fact that all these definitions and categories may change over time, and people of different ages or other demographic groups may use different vocabulary to describe similar behaviors or states of existence.

COLLECTING DATA ON GENDER IDENTITY

In broad population studies, data is usually gathered using a printed survey form, which may be filled out by the respondent or used by an interviewer to record data. Particularly if it is assumed the respondent will fill out the form without assistance (i.e., there is no interviewer who can answer questions or clarify meanings), the design of the form and the wording of the questions are of utmost importance. The researcher must be reasonably sure that all respondents will be able to read and understand the survey, that the questions and answers will mean the same things to each respondent, and that respondents will not be offended by the questions or the way they are worded. These issues are common to survey and questionnaire design, and there is a body of professional literature describing best practices and methods for creating survey instruments.

Collecting data on transgender people poses several particular issues, beginning with the wide range of terminology different people use to describe their gender identity. While it might seem like an obvious choice to simply ask "Are you transgender?" this question may confuse some respondents (e.g., many cisgender people are unfamiliar with the word *transgender* or mistakenly equate it with, homosexual behavior or orientation). It may also fail to capture information about respondents who might be included in a broad definition of transgender because they consider themselves to be, for instance, gender nonbinary, gender questioning, or simply the gender that they live on a daily basis. Certainly anyone studying minority sexualities would want to avoid falling into simple dichotomies— you're either cisgender or transgender—as surely as they would want to avoid asserting that there are only two genders, male and female, with no other possibilities allowed.

Choosing the right words is not a simple process, as researchers need to be sensitive to local norms in terminology and should test their survey form on representatives from the group to be surveyed, if possible. Making the time and effort to perform this step has the added advantage that the test subjects can inform the researchers if any part of the survey is unclear or offensive. The same guidelines apply if information about transgender status is to be collected for administrative rather than research purposes— the burden is on the people developing the form to understand the people who will be filling it out and to take special care to avoid confusion or offense.

While it might seem that the best solution is to simply allow free response, that is, allow each respondent to write in the words that they use to describe their gender identity, this poses problems when the data is analyzed. One reason for collecting demographic data (which also includes information such as an individual's race or ethnicity) is to be able to compare different groups (e.g., does job satisfaction differ between white and black Americans?) and a free response question may yield far too many categories to be useful. In addition, the data will need to be recoded if the data is to be analyzed statistically, and this requires extra man-hours while also offering the opportunity for errors and/or misinterpretation on part of whomever does the recoding.

Another possibility is to offer a list of descriptors (male, female, cisgender, transgender, gay, straight, etc.) and allow the respondents to check all that apply to them. While this may allow for collecting richer data that require individuals to select only one choice, it can also raise problems in analysis as the data may need to be recoded into combinations of characteristics. In addition, questions using lists are subject to biases such as the primacy effect (the first option may be chosen simply because it is the first), respondents may not read all the way to the end of the list, and some respondents may simply pick one answer and move on because they missed the instruction to check all that apply.

Multistep Questions

Two-step questions have been used to collect data about transgender individuals since at least the late 1990s. A simple example is the approach recommended by the Center of Excellence for Transgender Health in the Department of Family & Community Medicine at the University of California, San Francisco, for collecting gender identity information in medical practices. The first question asks, "What is your gender identity?" with five choices offered, plus the options to decline to answer or to write in a different word or phrase describing gender identity. The five options offered are male, female, transgender man/trans man, transgender woman/trans woman, and genderqueer/gender nonconforming. The second question asks, "What sex were you assigned at birth?" and offers the choices of male or female as well as the option to decline to answer. While the particular words used might vary from one community to another, the separation of current gender identity from gender assigned at birth allows the collection of far richer data than simply offering "transgender" as one option on a single question.

Greta R. Bauer and colleagues in Canada developed a three-step question to collect data about transgender identity. The first question asks the respondent to identify the sex they were assigned at birth, with the choices male or female. The second question asks the respondent to identify their current gender, offering four choices: male, female, "indigenous or other cultural gender minority identity (e.g., Two Spirit)" and "something else (e.g., gender fluid, nonbinary)". The third question asks the respondent to identify what identity they live in in their day-to-day life, with four choices offered: male; female; sometimes male, sometimes female; and "something other than male or female." This series of questions is appropriate for large surveys, because it can be processed entirely by computer (there are no free-response items), and the third question will only need to be answered by the subset of recipients (usually a small percentage of the total respondents) who indicate that their current gender identity does not match the sex they were assigned at birth.

One possibility that specifically captures information about the strength of identification as male or female is a multipart question that includes a scale with male at one end and female at the other. This type of question also has the advantage of specifically including those who identify as gender nonbinary and may yield interesting data about the strength of gender identity among individuals and how it correlates with other characteristics.

The Human Rights Campaign provides an example of a multipart question incorporating a visual scale in their youth survey. The first question asks the individual to indicate what gender they consider themselves to be, with check boxes for male, female, transgender, plus the possibility to write in a different answer. The second question is only for people who identified as transgender or other on the first question, and offers the choices male to female, female to male, neither, and other (with a blank to write the answer). The third question states that "Most people are born either male or female, but often feel or behave in a way that is different from what society believes is male or female behavior. One the scale below, please indicate either how male or female you feel" with a scale numbered from 0 (Male) to 10 (Female) (Human Rights Campaign, 2012).

SAMPLING

Gerald Sullivan and Warren Losberg discuss sampling methods and related issues with regard to studying LGBT individuals. While the mathematical aspects of sampling are well known, the common models of probability sampling (which aids the researcher's ability to generalize from the sample to the population) are less useful when studying sexual minorities.

There are many complex issues involved in sample-based research, but at heart the principle is that the researcher defines a population of interest, draws a sample from that population, and uses the results from the sample to make statements about the population. For instance, when a reputable polling firm announces that some percentage of Americans are in favor of this or that government policy, they have not contacted everyone in the United States and asked their opinion on the policy, but have drawn a sample scientifically and used results from the sample to generalize to the population. Both the definition of the population, and the way the sample is drawn, are crucial for the integrity of the results, and both are problematic in terms of studying transgender people.

The first issue is that of defining the population from which the sample may be drawn. While in some types of research this is a relatively simple matter (the population might be all persons in the United States aged 18 and older, e.g., or all men between the ages of 25 and 50 living in Detroit), even defining who is transgender raises difficulties. In addition, while demographic information such as age and race is regularly collected by governmental organizations such as the U.S. Census Bureau, so that we have a good idea of the racial makeup, for instance, of the population of the country, there is no similar national effort to collect information about gender and sexual identity. This means that answers to even such simple questions such as how many transgender people are currently living in the United States are not known.

The second problem involves drawing a sample from the population of interest. The best way to do this is through a probability sampling method, such as simple random sampling or stratified sampling. However, such methods are less useful when studying people with a rare characteristic such as transgender status, because a very large sample would need to be contacted to yield enough people with the characteristic to make the study practical (sufficient sample size is a basic requirement for accurate studies).

A third problem is that of collecting accurate information from the participants in a study. Even if a sample of sufficient size is collected by contacting people at random (e.g., through telephone surveys incorporating random digit dialing, with adjustments based on the fact that not everyone has a telephone or is willing to participate in a study), not everyone contacted may be willing to share information about their sexual or gender identity. In addition, the researcher and participant may not share a common definition of "transgender," making communication difficult. Those who are willing to disclose their transgender status with a researcher may be unrepresentative of the total population of transgender people, and thus the study will be based on a biased sample.

Many alternative survey designs using nonprobability samples are available, and much research has been conducted using these methods. Unfortunately, because these designs are generally not based on probability samples, the researcher's ability to generalize from the survey results is limit. One example of a nonprobability samples is the *snowball sample*, often used when studying groups that are otherwise difficult to locate. In this type of sample, current participants suggest future participants from among their acquaintances, giving researchers access to members of a group that might otherwise choose to remain hidden. Another type of nonprobability sample is the *convenience sample*, which as the name implies simply gathers data from those who are convenient to study. For instance, the researcher might interview people who were shopping in a popular mall on a Saturday afternoon, or those who choose to respond to a newspaper advertisement.

The problem with nonprobability samples, such as those drawn by using snowball or convenience sampling, is that the study participants are unlikely to be representative of the population which is the focus of the study. Such collection methods yield a sample, to be sure, but one which is most likely biased and thus from which no certain conclusions about the population as a whole can be drawn.

To put it another way, the study may accurately describe the people who participated in it, but there is no way to know whether the results of the sample apply to the larger population of interest. For instance, 40 percent of a convenience sample of transgender people may report being discriminated against at work, or 62 percent may say that they currently live with a romantic partner. Even assuming that those results are accurate in terms of the sample, there is no way to know from this information what percentage of the transgender population as a whole experience workplace discrimination or live with a romantic partner. Perhaps those who participated in the study were more or less likely to have those characteristics—with a nonprobability sample, we will never know.

Despite these difficulties, nonprobability sampling is not entirely useless. Methods such as snowball sampling are often used with groups who would otherwise not be studied at all because the population of interest is unlikely to identify themselves (snowball sampling has been used to study illicit drug users, for instance), and when information about a group is rare, any contributions may be useful. The point is to not become overenthusiastic in interpreting information from samples that were drawn in such a way that they cannot be used to generalize to a larger population. In addition, we can collect other information about participants in a study to see how they compare to those who did not participate—for instance, their race and ethnicity, which can be compared to data available from scientifically conducted surveys and censuses. Even if the demographics of a convenience sample exactly match those of a larger population, however, that cannot overcome the difficulties posed by generalizing from nonprobability samples.

STUDYING RACIAL AND ETHNIC MINORITY GROUPS

The problems of conducting research with transgender people may be compounded if the subjects are also members of racial and ethnic minority groups, particularly if the researcher does not come from the same racial or ethnic background. Darrell Wheeler suggests that self-awareness on the part of the researcher can go a long way toward creating productive research relationships, and that the first step researchers should take when conducting research within the African American GLBT community is to look critically at their own motives for wanting to conduct this research. He also suggests that researchers should think critically about their own beliefs concerns factors such as race, gender, and sexuality, and to also consider how their research will be used and what effect it may have on the research subjects and others similar to them. While it is impossible (and probably not desirable) to completely eliminate the fact that the researcher occupies an "other" role with respect to the research subject, awareness of this fact may also lead to more productive research relationships.

Wheeler also discusses practical issues involved with conducting research within the African American GLBT community, based on his own experience, and groups into five categories: confidentiality and the protection of human subjects; study design and the introduction of the study, sampling, instrumentation; and dissemination. While these issues are of concern to anyone doing social science research, they must be a particular focus for people studying people who have minority status both in terms of race and sexual or gender identification.

Confidentiality and protection of research subjects are principles that should be common to all social science studies; they are of particular concern when dealing with members of minority sexuality and minority racial and ethnic communities. Wheeler recommends consulting with one or more individuals from within the group to be studied, to help find culturally sensitive ways to specify the expectations and obligations of both researcher and research participant, and to frame the relationship between the two groups as more participative and inclusory than might be implied by the traditional researcher-subject paradigm.

Often, members of the community to be studied can make useful suggestions toward the design of a study. Even if the researcher chooses to not follow this path, he or she should be aware that the study may be perceived differently by the participants than by the researcher, and should be sensitive to how those perceptions may influence the results. In the case of transgender people and African Americans, participants have good historical reasons to be suspicious of researchers, and thus explaining the study in a non-patronizing manner is key to getting participants.

Sampling poses particular concerns among racial and sexual minorities, beginning with the fact that the definition of, say, who is African American, or who is transgender, differs among individuals. Understanding how such terms are understood within the community to be studied, and clarifying their use within the study, is necessary in order to produce meaningful results. In addition, the researcher must think of how other categories, such as economic status, may interact with the study's focus, and collect data on those factors, with an adequate sample in each category, allow for meaningful analysis.

In devising study instruments, such as questionnaires, the complexity of the subject and the perceptions of those within the studied group may be taken into account. For instance, gender or sexual identity may have many aspects, including self-perception, behavior, and the perception of others, and including all those aspects may lead to more meaningful research. In addition, the importance to an individual of, for instance, racial or ethnic identification, may vary, and these types of complexity require collection of much more information than simply checking off a racial descriptor from a set of categories.

Research without dissemination is analogous to the proverbial tree that falls in the forest where no one can hear it—if no one can read about the research and its results, the time and effort put into conducting the research has been wasted. Of course researchers are often most concerned with dissemination in the channels that will lead to professional recognition and advancement, but those may not be accessible to the community studies—articles may be behind paywalls and ideas expressed in obscure language—so particular effort should be made to inform participants and others in the community of the results of the research and to explain those results and field questions about them.

RESEARCH ETHICS

Transgender people are marginalized in American society, and many have experienced discrimination and violence because of their transgender status. In addition, sexual minorities have good reason to be suspicious of attempts by outsiders to study them. To take one well-known example in the field of sex research, the studies reported in the book *Tearoom Trade* by Laud Humphreys employed deceptive practices, failed to obtain informed consent from study participants, and failed to safeguard confidential information regarding study participants.

Without making any value judgments about transgender people, it is obvious that for some, revelation of their status could result in discrimination (e.g., in the workplace or in school), social ostracism (e.g., from family members), and perhaps expose them to violence. For these reasons, maintaining strong safeguards to protect the confidentiality of subjects, a basic requirement of most studies, is of particular importance when studying transgender people.

Researchers must also be aware of the influence study participation may have on the participants. For instance, someone who is unsure about their sexual or gender orientation might react strongly to being confronted with questions about their orientation during a survey. This problem might be addressed by including a full description of the study on the consent form, making psychological counseling available to study participants free of charge, or incorporating extensive debriefing procedures to help the study participants process their experience of participating in the study.

Researchers must also be aware of how the results of their study may be used by others. Even the most accurate results may have unintended consequences—for instance, data on sexual activity among transgender people might be distorted by a politician or journalist who wishes to portray such individuals as promiscuous and irresponsible. Presenting data with ample context (e.g., by providing data that compares the behavior of the studied group to others in the population) is one way to mitigate such risks. Another possibility is to consider at the time the study is being designed how the results could be used by those unfriendly to the group being studied, and to try to think of ways to prevent or counter such deliberate misinterpretation.

Anonymity is of particular concern to transgender people, and a number of methods have been developed to help protect this. For instance, if a questionnaire can be completed by the individual, either on paper or on a computer, with no identification that would link them to it, this may be preferable to even the best system of encryption. Methods in which a person flips a coin before deciding whether or not to answer a question truthfully also protect anonymity, and the results can be corrected for the incorporation of the coin flip when the data is analyzed. If identifying information (name, address, etc.) must be collected, it should be stored separately and securely from the study data, and linked through the use of anonymous IDs (e.g., numbers assigned to each participant, which could not be traced back to them without the use of the securely stored information). Bar codes can also be used to identify individuals, or they can be allowed to choose an ID number or name that they remember and use throughout the study.

Another ethical concern is ensuring that the subject understands what they are consenting to, a problem of particular concern when the subjects have a low degree of education or do not speak English as their first language. Any questionnaires used should be written at a reading level that the participants can easily understand, using vocabulary that will be familiar to them.

In the United States, persons younger than 18 years of age cannot give legal consent to participate in research. In terms of research, this is commonly interpreted as requiring the consent of the parent, as well as the minor participant, for any research study. In the case of transgender youth, this may pose a dilemma because the parent may be unaware of the child's transgender status, or disapprove of it. James I. Martin and William Meezan suggest several ways to work around these difficulties, including using independent advocates to safeguard the rights of study participants, or declaring the organization sponsoring the study to be acting *in loco parentis* for the purpose of the study (in any case, the minor must still consent to participate in the study).

PART III

Scenarios

CHAPTER 12

Case Studies

CASE STUDY 1: JANE

Jane is a six-year-old student in first grade at a public elementary school in a suburban area. She was identified as female at birth and has been raised as a girl. She attended kindergarten without incident and has displayed no issues in getting along with either her peers or adults. She is a bright child and in good health and has given no previous indication that she would have any adjustment issues. She is an only child and her parents are affluent and well-educated professionals, as are many of the parents of children who attend this elementary school. Jane's parents have provided a loving home for their daughter and want her to grow up healthy and happy.

The elementary school Jane attends is progressive and prides itself on not stereotyping children by gender. Students do not wear school uniforms and are allowed to dress comfortably within very general guidelines; for instance, many of the girls typically wear trousers or leggings rather than dresses or skirts. School staff make a conscious effort to refrain from gender policing and endeavor to prevent children from engaging in such activities. In particular, staff do not place limits or expectations on children's behavior based on their gender and avoid designating certain activities as appropriate for boys only and others as appropriate only for girls. For instance, both boys and girls are encouraged to play with both "boy toys" (e.g., trucks) and "girl toys" (e.g., dolls). Children of both genders are also encouraged to take part in both physical activities such as running and soccer, although the school tries to emphasize participation and the place of activity within a healthy lifestyle, rather than focusing on competition.

Although the school's general attitude is very inclusive and forward-looking, it has never had a transgender student before.

In the summer preceding her entry into first grade, Jane surprised her parents by asking that they call her "James" and insisted on getting a short haircut, rather than the ponytail she previous wore. (For the sake of clarity, this person will be referred to as "Jane" and by female pronouns, although as discussed later the counselor and parents should determine the child's preference for name and pronouns). While previously Jane had worn a variety of clothing, some of which would be coded as female in the United States, and some which would be coded as male, after declaring that she was a boy she only wanted to wear what her parents considered "boy's clothing"—t-shirts with logos of sports teams or male superhero characters, baseball caps, and so on. Jane also began insisting that she was not a girl but a boy, which baffled the parents because they had not received any prior indication that she was anything other than a girl who was happy to be a girl.

Although both parents are college educated and liberal on political and social issues, they have little knowledge of issues like sexual identity and are baffled that a child in a period of life, which they consider to be devoid of any sexual concerns, would have feelings and opinions on what seems to them to be a sexual matter. They are not prudish and assume that when their daughter reaches adolescence, she will become interested in boys, and that as a young adult one of her tasks in life will be to choose a marriage partner and form a family. Should she be romantically inclined toward other females, they are at least theoretically able to accept that choice as well. However, they did not anticipate that they would need to be dealing with what they consider a sexual issue while their daughter is so young.

Analysis

How might an elementary school guidance counselor respond in this situation? A guidance counselor plays many roles in the lives of the children who attend the school, and the adults who interact with them, and the specific actions that a counselor could take in this situation are partly guided by the counselor's own knowledge and expertise in transgender issues. One key task for the counselor in any case is to provide support for Jane and her parents, to help them understand their situation. A second is to see that the school provides the best possible experience for Jane, and to act as an advocate for Jane if there is resistance from within the school to making reasonable accommodations for her needs. The counselor can also refer Jane and her parents to resources in the community, which might include a physician and psychologist or counselor experienced in transgender issues, any support groups that may exist for parents and transgender children, and books and movies that explore the transgender experience, particularly the experiences of young transgender children and their families.

The counselor can also draw on his basic knowledge concerning gender identity in children and increase that knowledge through self-study and consultation with experts as necessary and feasible. An informed counselor can tell Jane's parents that it is not unusual for transgender children to make their first declarations of identity between ages 5 and 7, and that making such a declaration (e.g., Jane saying that she was a boy and choosing to adopt an appearance coded as male in American society) is not a matter of premature sexual knowledge but rather of felt gender identity. The counselor can assure the parents that there is no immediate need to make any decisions regarding matters like surgery or hormonal treatment, so they can support their daughter in her choices and see how things play out over the next few years. The counselor can tell them that many children who declare a transgender identity as young child do not persist in that identity as adolescents and adults, and that it is possible that at some point Jane will decide that she is a girl after all.

The counselor can inform the parents of the rights of all children to an appropriate education and can negotiate with the school staff to provide basic accommodations like referring to Jane by her preferred choice of name and pronouns. The counselor can also educate staff members and students by providing them with basic information about transgender children at a level appropriate to their understanding, and children can be coached in appropriate ways to interact with Jane. Specific issues like which restroom Jane will use and whether she will be considered a boy or a girl in sports (should that issue be relevant) can be determined through consultation with Jane and her parents, and the other students and staff educated about these decisions and the reasons for them. Above all, the focus should be on allowing Jane to complete her primary school education and develop her own sense of identity without imposing unnecessary restrictions on her.

Case Study 2: Sam

Sam is a middle-aged adult who was classified at birth as female but currently identifies as male and dresses and otherwise presents himself as male. One day he seeks care for abdominal pain at a medical clinic, giving his name to the intake clerk as "Sam" but presenting a driver's license that identifies him as female and with a different first name, although he looks a lot like the person in the license photo. He takes a clinic intake form and begins to fill it out; this form includes a choice of boxes to be checked to indicate whether the patient is male or female. Sam returns to the intake counter and confides in the intake clerk that he was identified as female at birth but now identifies as male and has lived as a man for the past five years. He has not changed his name or gender identity legally, however, and wants to know how he should fill out the intake form section requiring specification of gender. He seems somewhat nervous and ill at ease in the clinic setting, and also somewhat suspicious about why such a question would be necessary when he came to the clinic about a nonsexual matter.

The clinic is located in the downtown area of a large city. The patients who come to the clinic are diverse, but many are impoverished and many would be considered "outsiders" or "outlaws" in regard to conventional society—drug addicts, sex workers, sexual minorities, and so on. Many have no other medical home and rely on the clinic for whatever treatment they need. Many are uninsured or covered by Medicaid or Medicare, but the policy at the clinic has always been to attempt to provide care for everyone who asks for it and making referrals for those who need more specialized care.

The office staff of the medical clinic are a diverse group, representing many age groups, ethnicities, and political and social beliefs, while the medical staff is a mix of young professionals who have just started their careers and more experienced physicians and nurses, some of whom have worked there for years and see their work at the clinic as a way to make a positive difference in the world. However, not all of either the office or medical staff are well-informed on issues like gender identity and some harbor misconceptions common in the general population, such as confusing transgender identity with homosexuality or thinking of gender transition as primarily a matter of having surgery and taking hormones. Some are socially conservative and uncomfortable with matters such as minority sexualities (homosexuality, bisexuality, etc.) and divergent sexual identities (transgender, gender fluid, etc.).

Analysis

What could an intake clerk at a medical clinic do in this situation? The first thing the clerk should do is consider his assigned role in the process of providing care to Sam and all the other people who come to the clinic for care. Although that role is essentially bureaucratic, consisting primarily of handling paperwork, the clerk is also the first person a patient sees at the clinic, and thus the clerk's choices in terms of how to address the patients (e.g., with respect and using the name and pronouns preferred by the patient), thus communicating to the patient that he or she is valued and will be treated with respect by both the clerical and medical staff.

The clerk in this clinic plays another key bureaucratic role, that of assigning each new patient to a physician based on who is in the clinic and has room in their schedule that day. So while the clerk must remember that he or she is not a medical professional and thus is not qualified to provide medical advice, he or she does have the knowledge of different physicians, their expertise and attitudes, and can help Sam by assigning him to a physician familiar with transgender issues or at least lacking in prejudice against transgender people. The clerk is also responsible for being aware of laws such as HIPAA governing the confidentiality of patient records, and should assure Sam that his information is secure and will not be shared with anyone without his permission.

The clerk could tell Sam that the intake form should really include more than two categories for gender and/or allow patients to indicate their gender in their own words, and ideally would collect information both about gender as identified at birth and current gender identity. The clerk could add that realistically he or she can't change the existing form on the spot, but will bring up the issue at a meeting or through other appropriate channels. When doing so, the clerk should also educate the office and medical staff as to why the system of collecting gender information is inadequate. With regard to the immediate issue, the clerk could tell Sam to leave that part of the form blank and continue filling out the rest of it, assure him that he can share information about his birth gender and current sexual identity directly with the physician who treats him, and that he can ask the physician for advice about filling out that part of the form or leaving it blank.

CASE STUDY 3: CHRIS

Chris, a 20-year-old university sophomore, was identified as male at birth, has male genitalia and secondary sex characteristics (facial hair, broad shoulders), and lived the first 18 years of his life as male. Since coming to the university, however, he has begun to identify as genderqueer and has identified himself as such to his friends. As part of this coming out process, he has publicly declared that he no longer accepts the gender binary notion that individuals are either male or female, with no overlap, middle ground, or other possibilities, but has not undertaken any formal proceedings to change his name, legal gender identity, or to get a student ID or driver's license reflecting his new identity.

Chris sometimes dresses in clothing that in the United States is coded as male (suits and bow ties, baggy jeans and t-shirts) and sometimes in clothing coded as female (dresses, leggings, skirts). On his "female" days, he wears female-coded makeup, and on "male" days he wears no makeup. He lives in an off-campus private apartment but is frequently on the university campus for classes, social events, and to use resources like the library and computer center.

The university has not provided gender neutral restrooms for the students or staff, so all available restrooms are specifically designated for either males or females. Chris is in the habit of using the restroom that corresponds with his felt gender identity on the day in question, so if he feels male on a given day he will use the male restrooms, while if he feels female he will use the female restrooms. On a day that he felt female, Sam used one of the female restrooms on campus, and a female student using the restroom at the same time complained about him to the police officer. Chris's facial hair and male physique made her suspicious, and when she asked him if he was a man, he replied with a speech about why the gender binary is inadequate to describe the infinite variety of human beings, which she did not find at all amusing.

Although neither the city nor the state in which the university is located currently has a "bathroom bill" requiring people to use the public restroom that corresponds with their gender as assigned at birth, it is a fairly conservative area and most residents are not particularly well informed about transgender issues or concepts like gender fluidity. The student who made the complaint is sufficiently upset that she might take the matter to the city police if she feels the campus police do not take her seriously (Sam could be prosecuted for disturbing the peace or a similarly nonspecific crime). The campus police officer doesn't know what to make of a student with a beard who says he feels female, let alone one who says his gender identity changes from day to day. The only reason the police officer can imagine a male student would have for using the women's restroom involving being too drunk to tell the difference or being up to no good, perhaps planning to rob or molest women using that restroom. Nonetheless, the police officer hopes to bring the parties involved to some kind of reconciliation so that the matter can be settled without involving the city police.

Analysis

How could a psychologist at the student health clinic at Chris's university respond in this case? The psychologist in this case has never treated Chris, and in fact was unaware of his existence, so the counselor's role in this case will be to act as a mediator among the parties, to educate them about transgender and gender identity issues, and to inform both students about the psychological and counseling services available at the campus health center should they wish to take advantage of them. While the counselor may have personal opinions regarding the case (e.g., about who should use the women's restrooms on campus), she should serve here as a neutral party who hears the concerns of those involved and tries to help them come to some kind of understanding.

The counselor can validate Chris's choice to embrace a gender fluid identity, while also helping him appreciate how his appearance and behavior may be perceived by other students, faculty, and university staff. Without condemning his behavior, she can remind him that he shares the university with many people holding many different viewpoints, and from many different backgrounds, and that although the university setting allows him some freedom from the kind of behavioral restrictions and expectations typical in the "real world," such freedom is not absolute.

The counselor can sympathize with the student who made the complaint and reassure her that her feelings of shock upon seeing an apparent man in the woman's restroom are not illegitimate. She can further inform the student about transsexual and genderqueer issues, and help her appreciate the stress that accompanies the choice to live outside the usual gender categories of society. The counselor can also inform the student that while it may have been shocking to see what appeared to be a man in the women's bathroom, there are almost no cases of a man impersonating a woman to assault women in public restrooms, while gender nonconforming individuals face very real dangers of being attacked by men, in restrooms and elsewhere.

The counselor can educate the campus police officer on genderqueer and transsexual issues, helping him to see that Chris is working through issues of gender identity rather than sexuality, and is certainly not simply acting out in order to annoy conventional people. She can sympathize with the difficulty of his job, which involves trying to keep the peace among the diverse members of the university community, and with his desire to resolve the issue without the city police to becoming involved (if they do get involved, it might bring unwanted publicity to the university and discredit the campus police, among other things).

The ideal conclusion in this case requires that the counselor get each of the parties involved to see the situation from the point of view of the others, and to understand and appreciate those differing points of view. Chris needs to understand that not everyone around him embraces his views on gender and its expression, the complaining student needs to realize that her fears are not founded in reality and that Chris did not mean her any harm, and the campus police officer needs to realize that gender expression among young people is more varied than it may have been when he was young, but that is not necessarily a bad thing. While it is not necessary for the parties involved to embrace each other's point of view, in order to reach a satisfactory compromise they do need to appreciate that a variety of reasonable views exist on subjects as complex as gender identity and expression.

CASE STUDY 4: JOHN

John is a 30-year-old man who was classified as male at birth and was raised as a boy in a conservative, religious household. He grew up thinking that there were boys and there were girls, that each gender had specific roles to play in the world, and that was that. John began questioning his assigned gender identity in his early 20s, after moving away from home to attend university and then to accept a job as an engineer. He was a top student at his university and his parents were proud that he chose to study engineering, which they regard as an appropriate choice for a man. He is a valued employee at the large manufacturing corporation for which he works, where he presents himself as a man, but does not socialize much with his coworkers and has a reputation for keeping to himself. He has little social life outside work and is not married, nor is he currently interested in dating either men or women, in part because his greatest concern at the present moment is resolving his identity issues. His job provides him with a generous health insurance package, and should he decide to undergo gender transition most of his expenses would be paid for by his insurance plan.

Nothing in John's background prepared him to consider that he might be a transgender person, and he is not entirely clear about what the transition process might entail, which parts are reversible and which are not, and so on. He has done some informal research on the subject, but some of what he has learned there is incorrect or simply out of date, such as equating changing gender identity with undergoing genital surgery, or that it is a universal requirement to live for a year as the gender you intend to transition to before beginning the transition process.

John is also concerned about what transitioning to female might mean for his career, since engineering is a male-dominated field and he has seen excellent female engineers treated poorly within the company, both in terms of salaries and promotions and in terms of the general social climate (e.g., his boss loves to tell sexist jokes, and he feels pressured to laugh along with the other members of his team). The company climate is also hierarchical and conservative, and he's not certain how accepting his coworkers would be of a transgender person in their midst. Since a large part of John's identity is wrapped up in being a successful engineer, and on a daily basis most of his contact with other people comes at work, he does not want to risk damaging his career or becoming an object of ridicule, nor does he want to risk being shut out of the casual socializing that takes place in his office.

Analysis

What role can an endocrinologist experienced in transgender care play in this case? An endocrinologist is a physician specializing in the endocrine system, the glands that produce hormones to regulation matters such as metabolism, growth and development, and hormone treatment is often part of an individual's gender transition/gender affirmation process. An endocrinologist who has treated transgender patients can serve as a vital expert in educating transgender people about their options and providing them with treatment. Because there are many aspects to transition, ideally anyone who helps people through this process has established a network of physicians and other experts (e.g., voice therapists) to whom patients can be referred for additional care.

Because this physician has many transgender patients, he has made his office welcoming to trans people. Staff have been trained to treat everyone with respect and to ask what name and pronouns each patient prefers, and the office provides two gender-neutral, single-user restrooms. The clinic intake form collects information about gender as assigned at birth (with a "decline to answer" option as well) as well as current gender identity (allowing individuals to specify their gender in their own words) and records their preference for name and pronouns.

This is John's first visit to the clinic, so part of what the physician will do is similar to what any physician would do with a new patient, including taking a detailed medical history, getting the patient's permission to access his medical records from any other physicians he may be seeing, and generally becoming familiar with the patient, his personal situation, and the reason he has come to seek care. The physician perceives that John is experiencing distress due to the conflict between his current gender identity and his gender as assigned at birth, but also that he is not well-informed about the transition process and the many options available to him and is not entirely clear about the concept of gender identity itself. The physician's first priority therefore is to get to help John learn about gender identity and the many different ways that people experience their gender, as well as the range of procedures that are available should he decide he wants to proceed with gender transition.

The physician can provide John with a referral to a psychiatrist who has worked successfully with many transgender individuals in the past, to help him clarify what his current situation is and what options are available to him. He assures John that there's no rush and he should take as much time as he needs to decide what he wants to do next, he should decide what is right for him, and that and a team of physicians and healthcare professionals are ready to support him through whatever steps are required to resolve his conflict between his assigned and felt genders. The physician can also provide John with a referral to a social worker who specializes in workplace discrimination, to help him clarify what rights he would have in the workplace should he choose to transition, and what he should be prepared for in realistic terms. Truth is always the best policy, so the physician can't deny that transitioning to female might hurt John's career and cause some people to avoid him, but can encourage John to learn as much as he can about the transition process and to consider all the possible consequences, both positive and negative, when deciding what he wants to do.

CASE STUDY 5: MADISON

Madison is 15 years old and a sophomore at a private comprehensive high school. She was identified as male at birth and lived her early life as a boy, but began questioning her gender identity a few years ago. At the start of this school year, she arrived wearing a girls' uniform and requested that she be addressed using female pronouns. She told the school guidance counselor that she felt she was a girl and intended to start living as one. Her parents are supportive although also somewhat baffled by this choice, and they are able to provide her with whatever medical and psychological care she may need. They can also afford legal representation if Madison wants to challenge any decision restricting her ability to take part in school activities as a girl. Madison has consulted with a physician who is knowledgeable about transgender issues but has not begun hormone treatment or any other physical aspect of transition.

The high school fosters an inclusive atmosphere that values the uniqueness of each student, and both staff and students have been supportive of Madison's choice to present as female. In her freshman year, she was a good student and got along well with both her fellow students and the teaching staff, and has continued to do well both academically and socially in her sophomore year. All students in this high school are required to take part in at least one sport per year (exceptions have been made in the past for those unable to do so for health or cultural reasons). In her freshman year, Madison played basketball for the boys team and was moderately successful at both activities. Now she wants to participate in that sport again, but on the girls team. The head coach of the girls basketball team (a woman) is concerned that allowing someone who has the body of a boy to compete against girls will be unfair due to physical advantages (Madison is already taller and stronger than any of the female players currently on the team, and the difference can be expected to increase over the next two years), and that Madison might unintentionally injure the female players due to her larger size and strength. The coach is also concerned that some parents might refuse to let their daughters play on the same team as a boy and that other schools will refuse to allow their girls team to play against a team that includes an individual they regard as a boy, so that if Madison is allowed to play on the girls team some or all of the other girls will be deprived of the opportunity to compete in their chosen sport.

Analysis

What can the director of athletics at the high school contribute to help resolve this situation? Participation in sport is a fraught issue for transgender youth and sports administrators, particularly for young people identified male at birth but whose gender identity is female. By adolescence, boys are beginning to enjoy significant physical advantages over girls in most sports, one reason separate teams are the rule for this age group (unlike, say, Little League, where boys and girls can compete for the same team).

The athletic director decides on a two-pronged approach. First, she contacts the office of the governing body for the league in which the high school competes, and the governing body for all high school sports in the state, to see what rules and policies currently exist regarding transgender players and if any cases similar to that of Madison have already been handled by either governing body. Second, she arranges a meeting with Madison and her parents to explain the results of this investigation and the concerns of the other parties involved, and suggest some compromises that could resolve an admittedly difficult situation.

In this meeting, the athletic director emphasizes that the issue of how to define who is male and who is female is a difficult one, and that even international bodies like the International Olympic Committee have struggled to devise rules to accommodate transgender individuals. She also points out that the tradition of separate boys and girls teams predates our modern understanding of transgender issues, and thus that Madison doesn't fit neatly into the assumptions behind the structure of high school sports competition. She tells Madison that she supports her decision to present as female, but also informs her and her parents that both the state high school athletic association and the league in which the school competes require students to compete on teams appropriate to their gender as identified at birth. You also mention the concerns of the basketball coach that Madison enjoys a physical advantage over the other girls and might injure them without meaning to. You also mention that if Madison plays on the girls team, some parents may refuse to allow their daughters to play, and some schools will refuse to play against the school team, so that many other girls may be deprived of the opportunity to play. The athletic director concludes by stating that she will support Madison in whatever decision she makes regarding sports participation, including offering whatever expertise and assistance she can lend should Madison and her parents decide to challenge the birth-gender rule in court.

GLOSSARY

AFAB: Assigned female at birth. Also known as DFAB (designated female at birth).

Affirmed gender: The gender by which a person wishes to be known; usually used when a person's gender identity does not match his or her gender assigned at birth.

Agender: A person who does not identify as either male or female; a person who identifies as agender may have an identity between male and female, beyond the male/female spectrum, or as genderless.

Aggressive: A term used primarily in African American and Hispanic communities to describe masculine-presenting lesbians.

Ally: Someone who helps advocate for the rights of a group of which he or she is not a member, for example, a cisgender person who advocates for the rights of transgender people.

AMAB: Assigned male at birth. Also known as DMAB (designated male at birth).

Androgyne: Someone whose gender identity is both male and female, or neither male or female; an androgyne may present as male, female, both, or neither.

Androgynous: Having both male and female characteristics.

Antiandrogen: Also known as an androgen blocker, a drug used to block the effects of androgens such as DHT; androgens are sometimes used by trans women undergoing gender reassign and have other medical uses as well (e.g., to treat prostate cancer).

Asexual: A person who does not have sexual desires or feelings. Asexuality is distinct from celibacy, which includes people who may have sexual feeling or desires but choose to not have sex.

Assigned sex/assigned gender: The sex/gender to which an individual is assigned at birth, usually based on external genitalia, which may or may not correspond to an individual's gender identity.

Berdache: A historical term now in disfavor referring to gender nonconforming individuals in Native American tribes. A more acceptable term is *Two Spirit*.

Binding: Constraining the breasts by use of cloth or elastic material in order to have a more male-appearing chest.

Biological sex: An individual's sex as determined by physical characteristics at birth, including genitalia and chromosomal makeup; biological sex may or may not correspond to an individual's gender identity.

Boi: A term sometimes used to describe a young transgender man, a genderqueer person, or a masculine woman.

Bottom surgery: Surgery on the external and/or external and internal genitalia and reproductive organs; examples include phalloplasty and vaginoplasty.

Breast augmentation: Surgery to make the breasts larger. Some trans women opt for breast augmentation surgery, while others find that hormone treatment produces sufficient breast growth.

Carry letter: A letter about an individual's trans status, provided by a medical professional, that some individual's use to facilitate communication with officials, for instance, while traveling or in case of interactions with police.

Cisgender: An individual who is not transgender, that is, one whose gender assigned at birth matches their gender identity.

Cisnormativity: The assumption that the usual, normal, or only acceptable state of affairs is for everyone's gender at birth to match their gender identity.

Cliteroplasty: Surgical creation of a clitoris.

Clocking: Also known as reading, identifying a person's gender as other than how they present themselves. For instance, an anatomical man dressed as a woman who is identified by a bystander as a man has been clocked/read.

Closeted: A term used to describe someone who is not open about their gender identity or sexual orientation.

Coming out: Sharing information about one's gender or sexual identity that is not otherwise known; for instance, informing someone of one's transgender status.

Cross-dressing: Wearing clothing associated with a gender other than that of the individual wearer; cross-dressing may or may not be indicative of transsexual status or other gender nonconformity.

DHT: Dihydrotestosterone, an androgen hormone.

Drag king: A person who dresses in masculine clothing and displays behaviors associated with men as part of a performance; drag kings are often, but not necessarily, individuals who were assigned female at birth (AFAB).

Drag queen: A person who dresses in feminine clothing and displays behaviors associated with women as part of a performance; drag queens are often, but not necessarily, individuals who were assigned male at birth (AMAB).

DSD: Disorders or differences of sex development, a term roughly equivalent to *intersex*, describing congenital conditions in which some aspect of an individuals' sex (anatomical, chromosomal, or gonadal) is atypical.

DSM: *The Diagnostic and Statistical Manual of Mental Disorders* of the American Psychiatric Association, a publication that is used to identify and classify mental disorders. The fifth and most recent edition is referred to as *DSM-5*. The *DSM* is highly influential and sometimes controversial; for instance, until 1973, homosexuality was included in the *DSM* as a mental disorder.

Electrolysis: A method of permanently removing hair from the body by destroying the hair follicles with electricity.

Elverson pronouns: A set of gender-neutral pronouns proposed by Christine Elverson in 1975; they include "ey" as a replacement for the subject pronouns "he" and "she," "em" as a replacement for the object pronouns "him" and "her" and "eir" as a replacement for the possessive adjectives "his" and "her."

Estrogen: A sex hormone responsible for the development of the female reproductive system and secondary sex characteristics; both men and women have some amount of estrogen naturally, but women typically have a greater amount.

FFS: Facial feminization surgery, surgery intended to make a person's face more typically feminine in appearance. Examples include contouring the forehead, rhinoplasty (nose surgery), and chin reduction.

FTM: Female to male, that is, someone who was assigned female gender at birth but identifies as male.

GAS: Gender-affirming surgery, also known as GCS or gender-confirming surgery, GAS is surgery to help a person's body match their gender identity. Other related terms include *sexual reassignment surgery* and *genital reconstruction surgery*.

Gay-straight alliance: A student-run club for gay, lesbian, transgender, and other gender nonconforming students, their allies, and questioning people. The aims of a Gay-straight alliance aims typically include providing a safe space for students to meet and talk about issues related to gender identity and sexuality, providing support for members and other gender nonconforming people, and to take social and political action.

GD: Gender dysphoria, a term used in *DSM-5* (the fifth edition of the American Psychiatric Association's *Diagnostic and Statistical Manual of Mental Disorders*) to describe an experienced and marked incongruence between a person's assigned gender and their gender identity. The previous term for this condition was *GID* or *gender identity disorder.*

Gender: A set of traits, which may include social, psychological, and emotional factors that classify someone as male, female, or neither.

Gender bender: A self-identification of a person who believes the categories of "male" and "female" do not adequately describe them; a gender bender may present themselves as male, female, both, or neither.

Gender binary: The belief that only two genders, male and female, exist, and that every person must be one or the other.

Gender expansive: A term broadly used to describe people whose gender identity is not limited to gender norms for their society; a gender expansive person's

identity may be beyond binary male/female notions, between the two genders, or otherwise not conform to societal norms.

Gender expression: External signs of gender, such as voice, name, clothing, and
mannerisms, used consciously or unconsciously, which communicate one's
gender to others. Whether a particular gender expression is classified as male
or female or neither is a matter of culture, and not all cultures agree on these
classifications.

Gender identity: A person's sense of their own gender, whether male, female, or
something else; gender identity may or may not correspond to the gender an
individual is assigned at birth. For other people, their gender identity may not
match or fit neatly into either the category of male or female. Gender identity
is a personal sense and is not visible to other people.

Gender minority: An individual whose gender identity or gender expression
does not conform to the expectations of their society or culture.

Gender neutral: Not assigned to one gender or the other; for instance, a gender
neutral bathroom can be used by anyone.

Gender nonconforming: An adjective describing people whose gender expression does not match the norms in their culture for masculinity and femininity. While there may be overlap between gender nonconforming people and
transgender people, the terms are not synonymous, and gender nonconformity does not make a person transgender.

Gender norms: Expectations about how people are supposed to look or behave,
based on their gender.

Gender policing: The monitoring of other people's behavior, based on the beliefs
or expectations about gender norms of the person doing the policing, and the
attempt to impose gender norms on other people.

Gender spectrum: The context that gender exists on a continuum rather than a
male/female dichotomy; an individual may identify at any point on the spectrum, off the spectrum entirely, or move fluidly about the spectrum.

Genderqueer: A self-identification used by some people who feel that their gender expression and/or gender identity fits neither the male or female categories offered by their culture.

GLAAD: An organization formerly known as the Gay and Lesbian Alliance
against Defamation, which was founded in 1985 in response to sensation-
alized coverage of HIV and AIDs in the *New York Post*. GLAAD monitors
media reports for defamation of gay, lesbian, and transgender people, provides guidelines for reporting and discussing GLBT people and issues, and
bestows annual awards for outstanding presentations of GLBT issues and
characters in both news/factual and creative media (the latter including,
among other things, movies, television, and novels).

GnRH analogues: Gonadotropin-releasing hormone analogue, a drug taken
to delay the onset of puberty by suppressing production of estrogen or
testosterone.

HBSOC: The Harry Benjamin Standards of Care, a set of guidelines for medical
and mental health professionals who treat transgender people.

Hermaphrodite: An historical term, sometimes considered derogatory, referring to people who have characteristics of both gender.

Heteronormativity: The assumption that heterosexuality is the normal or only acceptable type of gender identity.

Hir: A gender neutral pronoun that can be used in place of the gendered third-person pronouns "him" and "her."

Homophobia: Fear or dislike of lesbian and gay people.

Hormone: A chemical substance produced by glands in the body; hormones regulate physiology and behavior.

HSO: Hysterectomy and salpingo-oophorectomy: Surgery to remove the uterus, ovaries, and fallopian tubes; HSO is sometimes performed to treat or prevent cancer as well as during bottom surgery for gender transition.

"I AM: Trans People Speak": A campaign created by the Massachusetts Transgender Political Coalition to create awareness of transgender people and communities. "I AM" consists of videos by transgender people and their families, friends, and allies.

Intersectionality: A concept in sociology describing how different social systems and forms of oppression may interact; for instance, an individual may be oppressed by both gender bias and racial discrimination.

Key population: In public health research, a group that is at particular risk for some disease or condition. For instance, transgender people are a key population in HIV risk, because they are at higher risk to be infected with HIV.

Labiaplasty: Bottom surgery in which the labia is created or enhanced.

Mastectomy: Surgical removal of the breasts, a type of top surgery sometimes performed as part of the transition process.

Metoidioplasty: A type of bottom surgery in which the clitoris is separated from the labia minora and the suspensory ligament is cut, to allow the clitoris to assume a lower position similar to that of the penis. Metoidioplasty is usually performed in conjunction with testosterone replacement therapy to enlarge the clitoris.

Misgender: To refer to someone by a pronoun or other term that does not reflect their gender identity; for instance, referring to a transgender woman as "he."

MSM: Men who sleep with men, a term used in public health and medicine to identify people based on their sexual practices (e.g., when evaluating the risk for certain diseases) rather than gender or sexual identity.

MTF: Male to female, a person who was assigned male gender at birth but identifies as female.

Mx: Also written as "Mixter," a gender-neutral title that can be substituted for "Mr.," "Mrs.," and "Miss."

Natal sex: The sex a person was assigned at birth, which may or may not correspond to their sense of gender identity.

Nonbinary: A self-identification used by people who don't feel that either "male" or "female" adequately defines them.

Oophorectomy: Surgical removal of the ovaries.

Orchiectomy: A type of bottom surgery in which the testicles are removed.

Outing: Revealing information about someone's sexual orientation or gender identity without the permission of that person.

Packing: Wearing an object in one's underwear or trousers to make it appear that one has a penis.

Passing: For a transgender person, to be perceived by strangers as the gender one identifies with. Some people find the term pejorative because it implies that one can fail at performing gender.

Penectomy: A type of bottom surgery in which the penis is removed.

PGP: Preferred gender pronouns, the pronouns a person prefers to be addressed by (he, she, ze, etc.).

Phalloplasty: A type of bottom surgery in which a penis is created.

Puberty blockers: Also called puberty suppressors, drugs used to delay the onset of puberty.

Questioning: A term used to describe people who are exploring or discovering their gender or sexual identity, orientation, or expression.

Real-life experience: A period of time when persons planning on gender transition live as their identified gender, before beginning surgical or hormonal treatments.

Salpingectomy: Surgical removal of the fallopian tubes.

Scrotoplasty: Bottom surgery that creates a scrotal sack.

Secondary sexual characteristics: Body characteristics such as the pitch of the voice, hair on the face and body, and changes in the breasts and hips, which develop at puberty and are associated with being male or female.

Sex change: A term formerly used for what is now usually called gender-affirming surgery or gender-confirming surgery; the latter terms are preferred because many individuals believe their sex or gender is not changed as a result of the surgery, but that the surgery is bringing their body into line with what has always been their sex or gender.

Sexual orientation: A person's physical, emotional, or romantic attraction toward another. Gender identity and sexual orientation are separate issues, and a transgender person may be heterosexual, bisexual, lesbian, or gay.

Social construction of gender: A sociological idea that gender roles, including behaviors deemed appropriate for males and females, are societal and cultural constructions rather than being the inevitable result of biological factors.

Spivak pronouns: A set of gender-neutral pronouns proposed by the mathematician Michael Spivak. Spivak pronouns including "e" replacing the subject pronouns "he" and "she," "em" replacing the object pronouns "him" and "her," and "emself" replacing the reflexive pronouns "himself" and "herself."

STD: A sexually transmitted disease, that is, a disease that can be transmitted through sexual contact. Examples include HIV/AIDS, syphilis, chlamydia, herpes, and hepatitis B.

STI: A sexually transmitted infection, that is, an infection that can be transmitted through sexual contact. Some people prefer the term *STI* to *STD*, because sometimes STIs do not cause disease symptoms.

Stealth: Choosing to not reveal one's transgender status.

STP device: A device allowing a person to urinate while standing (when it would otherwise not be possible for that person); the letters stand for "stand to pee."

Tanner scale: Also called the Tanner stages, a scale of physical development based on primary and secondary sex characteristics. One use of the Tanner scale is to determine the onset of puberty, and thus for a transgender child, when to begin using puberty-delaying drugs.

TDOR: The Transgender Day of Remembrance, founded by transgender advocate Gwendolyn Ann Smith and celebrated on November 20 of each year to honor the memory of the transgender woman Rita Hester (killed in 1998) and all transgender people killed by violence.

TGNC: Trans and gender nonconforming.

Third sex: Also called third gender, a term for people who identify as neither male nor female.

Top surgery: Surgery changing the appearance of one's chest, to match one's gender identity. For female-to-male transgender people, top surgery typically involves a mastectomy (surgical removal of the breasts), while for male-to-female transgender people, top surgery may include breast implants.

Tracheal shave: Also known as chrondrolaryngoplasty, a surgical technique that reduces the size of the Adam's apple by shaving down the thyroid cartilage.

Trans man: A transgender person whose identity is male.

Trans woman: A transgender person whose identity is female.

Transgender: An umbrella term used to refer to people whose gender identity does not correspond with their sex assigned at birth, or whose gender expression is not congruent with societal norms. Many people argue that "transgender" should only be used as an adjective, not a noun, so "he is a transgender man" is preferable to "he is a transgender."

Transgender Awareness Week: A week in November devoted to raising awareness about transgender and gender nonconforming people; Transgender Awareness Week ends with the Transgender Day of Awareness (TDOR), which commemorates transgender people killed by violence.

Tranny chaser: A person who seeks out the company or affections of, or desires sexual activity with, transgender people. Many people find the term derogatory and insulting to both transgender people and the "chasers."

Transition: The process of changing from the sex assigned at birth. The particular steps involved in transition vary from one person to the next, but may include informing people of the change; using a different name and/or different pronouns for self-reference; changing one's style of dress; changing legal documents; having surgery; and undergoing hormone treatment.

Transphobia: Fear or dislike of people who do not confirm to gender roles expected by the individual who is transphobic.

Transsexual: An older term used to refer to people who have made permanent changes to their bodies, for instance, through surgery or hormone treatment;

some argue that "transsexual" should only be used as an adjective ("a trans-sexual man").

Transvestite: A person who wears clothing associated in their culture with the opposite sex, as a form of gender expression (not for purposes of entertainment).

Two spirit: A term used to describe people who believe they have "two spirits in the same body," that is, a mix of male and female spirits such that they correspond to a third gender rather than to either male or female. In some cultures, the term *Two Spirit* does not signify being a transgender person. *Two Spirit* is also a preferred term to replace the term *berdache* when discussing some Native American cultures.

Vaginoplasty: A type of bottom surgery in which a vagina is created, typically by using skin from the penis.

Ze: A gender-neutral pronoun that can replace "he" and "she."

Zir: A gender-neutral pronoun that can be used in place of the gendered third-person pronouns "him" and "her."

Timeline

1629	Thomas/Thomasine Hall, in what is now the state of Virginia, claims to be both male and female. A judge agrees and Hall is ordered to wear articles of clothing customarily identified with both men and women.
1652	In what is now New Hampshire, Joseph Davis is fined for the crime of wearing clothing associated with women.
1738	Esther Brandeau, a French Jewish woman disguised as a Catholic male sailor (using the name "Jacques La Fargue"), arrives in Canada; when her gender and religion are discovered, she is deported back to France.
1782	Deborah Samson serves in the Continental Army during the American Revolutionary War by passing as a man.
1812	Transgender man James Barry graduates from medical school and goes on to work as an army surgeon and hospital administrator; his birth sex becomes publicly known only after his death in 1865.
1848	Columbus, Ohio, outlaws cross-dressing; many other cities pass similar laws in the coming years, including Chicago in 1851, Newark, New Jersey, in 1858, and San Francisco, California, in 1863.
1861–1865	During the American Civil War, a number of individuals (some historians estimate over 200) serve as male soldiers, although they were assigned at birth to the female gender.
1864–1865	Austrian physician Karl Heinrich Ulrichs publishes *Researches on the Riddle of "Man-Manly" Love*, a series of pamphlets positing a theory of same-sex attraction based

on the concept of "a female soul within a male body"; he coined the term *urning* to refer to such individuals.

1869   German psychiatrist Karl Friedrich Otto Westphal publishes the first medical paper describing transgender people.

1878   After her death, a person known as "Mrs. Nash," who had married several men and worked as a laundress for George Custer, is discovered to have the body of a man.

1879   American Lucy Ann Lobdell/Joseph Lobdell is confined to the Willard Insane Asylum in New York. Lobdell was assigned female at birth but considered herself a man; some modern historians classify Lobdell as a transgender person, others as a lesbian.

1883   The first use of the term *lesbian*, to describe the transgender man Joseph Lobdell, who lived as a man but was assigned female gender at birth (his birth name was Lucy Ann Lobdell).

1899   German physician Magnus Hirschfeld begins publishing the *Yearbook for Sexual Intermediaries*, the first scientific journal devoted to the study of minority sexualities; the journal continues publication until 1923.

1901   New York City politician Murray Hall dies from breast cancer and is discovered to have the body of a woman; he had lived as a man and may have avoided medical care in order to protect his secret.

1910   German physician Magnus Hirschfeld coins the term *transvestite*.

1917   Alan L. Hart, an American physician, becomes one of the first people known to under transition from male to female in the United States. Hart, born as Lucille Hart in 1890, had a hysterectomy and gonadectomy, and lived the remainder of his life as a man.

1918   Publication of *The Autobiography of an Androgyne* by Jennie June, a transgender woman who was born in Connecticut as Earl Lind.

1919   German physician Magnus Hirschfeld founds the Institut für Sexualwissenschaft (Institute for Research into Sexuality) in Berlin. It is destroyed by the Nazi regime in 1933.

1930   The Danish painter Lili Elbe, born Einar Wegener, becomes the first person known to undergo male-to-female sexual reassignment surgery; she died after surgery to implant a uterus in her body.

1931   Dora Richter undergoes male-to-female surgery, including genital transformation; the surgery is arranged by Magnus Hirschfeld.

1937	American surgeon Hugh Hampton Young publishes *Genital Abnormalities, Hermaphroditism*, and Related Adrenal Disease, which describes genital surgery on intersexual patients.
1939	The touring drag show *The Jewel Box Revue* begins performing at the Club Jewel Box in Miami.
1941	The Langley Porter Psychiatric Clinic is founded at the University of California, San Francisco; it becomes a major center for research into sexual and gender minorities.
1947	John Herbert is arrested in Toronto for being dressed as a woman. He will later draw on his experiences of incarceration in a youth detention center in his 1967 play *Fortune and Men's Eyes*, which was made into a film in 1971.
1949	Robert Latou Dickinson publishes *Human Sex Anatomy*, which uses the term *intersex*, discusses ambiguous genitals on a continuum rather than as discrete categories, and includes illustration of ambiguous genitalia.
1948	German-American physician Harry Benjamin treats the first of many patients with hormone therapy; his initial patient is a boy who wants to be a girl.
1948	American scientist Alfred Kinsey publishes *Sexual Behavior in the Human Male*, which includes the "Kinsey Scale," also known as the "Heterosexual-Homosexual Rating Scale." This scale describes a person's sexual orientation on a scale from 0 (exclusively heterosexual) to 6 (exclusively homosexual). Kinsey follows-up in 1953 with publication of *Sexual Behavior in the Human Female*.
1952	Christine Jorgensen, an American who had male-to-female gender affirming surgery in Denmark, becomes the first widely known transgender person. Although Jorgenson was not the first individual to have gender-affirming surgery, her celebrity status (Jorgenson's story was front-page news, and she worked as an actress and entertainer following her surgery) raised awareness of transgender people.
1952	Publication of the journal *Transvestia: The Journal of the American Society for Equality in Dress*, founded by the transgender woman Virginia Price; only two issues are published.
1952	In Los Angeles, the self-described homophile publication *ONE* magazine begins publishing and is the first publication supporting gay rights to be sold at newsstands. A federal district court temporarily banned *ONE* from mail distribution due to obscenity, but in 1958 the U.S. Supreme Court overturned this decision.

May 1959	Patrons of Cooper's Donuts, a popular hangout for transgender and LGBT people in Los Angeles, respond to police attempts to arrest a trans woman by causing a minor riot; the following day, the restaurant is picketed.
1962	The Gender Identity Research Clinic is founded at UCLA.
1963	John Rechy publishes *City of Night*, a novel describing the experiences of a young man working as a sexual hustler in the United States; some of the characters, including one called "Miss Destiny," might be described today as transgender people, although that terminology did not exist at the time.
1964	Reed Erickson, a trans man, founds the Erickson Educational Foundation to promote lesbian, gay, bisexual, and transgender equality.
1965	A number of gender nonconforming individuals are arrested after refusing to leave Dewey's Coffee Shop in Philadelphia, which had a policy of not serving people wearing "nonconformist" clothing. The shop changed its policy after being picketed by the GLBT community.
1966	German-American physician Harry Benjamin publishes *The Transsexual Phenomenon*, describing his work with transgender patients. This book included the Sexual Orientation Scale, which classified different types of transvestism and transsexualism (using the terms in use at the time) in men.
1966	The first American legal case involving transgender status is heard in New York State: *Mtr. Of Anonymous v. Weiner* ("Weiner" was Louis Weiner, then director of the Bureau of Records and Statistics of the Department of Health for the city of New York). The case involved the request of an individual to have the sex designated on his/her birth certificate to be changed from male (as assigned at birth) to female (the individual's gender identity). The Department of Health refused to make the change, although the individual in question had undergone what was then called sex reassignment surgery, and the court upheld the department's decision, stating that the law allowed only the sex on a birth certificate to be changed if an error was made when it was recorded in the first place.
1966	New Zealand-American physician John Money opens the Gender Clinic at Johns Hopkins. It champions gender reassignment surgery, but its reputation is later tainted by revelations that important facts about one of Money's early patients, David Reimer, who was born male but underwent gender reassignment to female, were fabricated.

August 1966	In San Francisco, California, police attempt to arrest a transgender patron of Compton's Cafeteria results in a riot; the Compton's Cafeteria Riot is now considered a landmark in the evolution of transgender rights.
1967	Founding of the first known organization for transsexuals, COG, in San Francisco. The acronym has been identified as standing for either Change: Our Goal or Conversion Our Goal. COG worked to increase public knowledge about transsexuality and to help individuals who wanted sex reassignment surgery get access to it.
1967	The Polish runner Ewa Klobukowska becomes the first person to be banned from competing as a woman, after failing a chromosome test. She had mosaic XX/XXY chromosomes, and ironically would have been classified as a woman in the 1968 Olympics, when a different method (the Barr Body test) was used to determine who would qualify as female.
1968	The International Olympic Committee requires female athletes to undergo chromosome testing at the Mexico City Summer Olympics, based in part on the suspicion that some Russian and Eastern European athletes competing as female are in fact male. The test in use at the time, which was based on the SRY (sex-determining region Y) protein, was later abandoned as inconclusive.
June 28, 1969	Following arrests, patrons of the Stonewall Inn in New York City, a club which was patronized by many gay, lesbian, and transgender people, the patrons and others gathered outside begin a riot that requires the police to take refuge within the club. The Stonewall Riots were followed by demonstrations and organizing, including creation of the Gay Liberation Front, and are considered by many historians to be the birth of the modern gay rights movement.
1970	In Great Britain, the marriage of April Ashley and Arthur Cameron Corbett is annulled because Ashley was assigned to the male gender at birth.
1970	Opening of STAR (Street Transvestite Action Revolutionaries) House in New York City, by Silvia Rivera and Marsha P. Johnson; STAR house offers shelter and support to young transsexuals.
1970	Founding of Transsexual Action Organization by Angela Keyes Douglas in California.
October 21, 1971	Opening of Lee's Mardi Gras Boutique, a shop in New York City serving drag performers and cross-dressers; it was founded by Lee Greer Brewster, a drag queen and transgender activity.

1972	Sweden legalizes gender affirmation surgery, making it the first country in the world to do so.
1972	The British writer Jan Morris, born James Morris, transitions from male to female; she writes about her experiences as a transgender person in the 1974 memoir *Conundrum*.
1972	The San Francisco chapter of the lesbian organization Daughters of Bilitis votes to exclude transgender women.
1972	"Walk on the Wild Side," a song written and performed by Lou Reed, includes references to transsexuality, including the transgender women Holly Woodlawn, Candy Darling, and Jackie Curtis, all "superstars" associated with Andy Warhol and his circle.
1973	Trans woman Beth Elliot becomes vice president of the lesbian organization Daughters of Bilitis but is forced to resign by members who thought the organization should only include those assigned female gender at birth.
1974	Founding of Howard Brown Health in Chicago, an organization providing health care and social services to gay, lesbian, bisexual, and transgender people.
1975	Minneapolis becomes the first city in the United States to pass a law guaranteeing transgender people protection from discrimination.
1975	Sidney Lumet's film *Dog Day Afternoon* includes a transgender character in a small role that is crucial to the plot. The central character, played by Al Pacino, robs a bank in order to pay for his lover's gender reassignment surgery.
1975	A Connecticut court rules in *Darnell v. Lloyd* that if the state refuses to change the sex recorded on an individual's birth certificate upon request, the state must demonstrate substantial interest in refusing the request.
1976	Renee Richards, a trans woman born Richard Raskind, is denied the right to compete as a woman in a tennis tournament.
1977	The New York Supreme Court rules that the transgender woman Renee Richards has the right to compete as a woman in tennis.
1977	The Oregon Supreme Court rules in *K. v. Health Division* that there is no legislative authority to allow an individual's name or sex to be changed on a birth certificate based on the individual's transgender status.
1978	*In a Year of 13 Moons*, a film by the German director Rainer Werner Fassbinder, features a character who undergoes male-to-female sexual reassignment surgery.

1978	The rainbow flag, which has become a well-known symbol of gay, lesbian, bisexual, and transgender pride, is first displayed as part of the Gay Freedom Day parade in San Francisco.
October 14, 1979	The first National March on Washington for Lesbian and Gay Rights is held in Washington, DC; one of the organizers, Phyllis Frye, later became the first openly transgender person to be appointed as a judge in Texas.
1979	The Harry Benjamin International Gender Dysphoria Association is founded; one of the group's accomplishments is to create standards for the diagnosis and treatment of people whose gender identity does not match the gender they were assigned at birth.
1980	In Great Britain, the Self Help Association for Transsexuals is founded; the organization's name is later changed to the Gender Dysphoria Trust International.
1980	The term *transsexualism* is added to the third edition of the *Diagnostic and Statistical Manual of Medical Disorders* (*DSM-III*) published by the American Psychiatric Association. In later editions, the term *gender identity disorders* is used instead.
1980	In Germany, transgender people are allowed to change their legal gender, although they must have undergone genital surgery in order to do so.
1980	Founding of the ACLU Transsexual Rights Committee in Southern California; one of this organization's achievements was the creation of separate wings in California state prisons for preoperative transgender people.
1982	John Lithgow, a cisgender man, is nominated for an Academy Award for his portrayal of a transgender man Roberta Muldoon in *The World According to Garp*.
1982	Cisgender actress appears as a transgender woman from a small Texas town in Robert Altman's film *Come Back to the Five & Dime, Jimmy Dean, Jimmy Dean*; the film is based on a play by Ed Graczyk.
1982	Founding of the Educational TV Channel in San Francisco. Originally primarily focused on providing support to male-to-female cross-dressers, it later expanded to include transgender people and changed its name to TransGender San Francisco.
1984	In *Ulane v. Eastern Airlines Inc.*, the Seventh Circuit Court denies the claim that Karen Ulane, who was assigned male gender at birth and transitioned to female in 1980, was being

fired based on her having undergone sex reassignment surgery constituted discrimination against women.

1984   Founding of the Harvey Milk High School in New York City. Named after the assassinated gay San Francisco politician, it is the first public school created specifically to serve gay, lesbian, bisexual, and transgender students.

1985   Founding of the media-monitoring organization GLAAD (formerly known as the Gay & Lesbian Alliance against Defamation), in part due to sensationalizing coverage of the HIV/AIDS crisis by the *New York Post*. GLAAD changed its name to signal that its scope also included transgender and bisexual issues.

1986   Lou Sullivan founds FTM in San Francisco; it is the older organization established specifically for transgender men.

1987   The 1987 revision of the *Diagnostic and Statistical Manual* of the American Psychiatric Association, known as *DSM-III-R*, adds the classification "gender identity disorder."

1987   Founding of the International Foundation for Gender Education in Massachusetts.

1989   Death of Billy Tipton, a transgender man born in Oklahoma as Dorothy Lucille Tipton. Tipton was a jazz piano player and bandleader who used a male persona when performing; his birth sex was discovered when he was treated at a hospital for an ulcer, and many stories about his transgender status appeared in news sources after his death.

1990   Jennie Livingston's documentary *Paris Is Burning*, which chronicles ball culture in New York City, brings broad public awareness to this aspect of the transgender and gay Latin American and African American community. *Paris Is Burning* won numerous awards, including a Grand Jury Prize from the Sundance Film Festival and a Teddy Bear from the Berlin International Film Festival, but was not nominated for an Academy Award, a result that helped bring about change in the way the documentary awards were handled by the Motion Picture Academy.

1990   The American Educational Gender Information Service (AEGIS), which provides transgender education and resources, is founded in Atlanta by Dallas Denny. From 1990 to 1998, AEGIS published *Chrysalis Quarterly*.

1991   Transgender woman Nancy Burkholder is removed from the Michigan Womyn's Music Festival, a woman-only event. As a result, transgender women and their allies began holding a demonstration and event known as Camp Trans outside the Festival each year.

1991   The first Southern Comfort Conference is held in Atlanta; it features speeches, seminars, events, and vendors relevant to transgender people.

1992   *The Crying Game*, a film by the British director Neil Jordan, includes a transgender character in a key role.

1993   Brandon Teena, a trans man, was murdered in Humboldt, Nebraska; Teena's death heightened awareness of hate crimes against transgender people, while his story informed the 1999 feature film *Boys Don't Cry*, where Teena was played by the cisgender actress Hilary Swank.

1993   Cheryl Chase founds the Intersex Society of North America. The organization's goals include informing the public about intersex people and advocating for an end to unnecessary surgeries on intersex people.

1993   Cisgender actress Olympia Dukakis stars in the television production of *Tales of the City* as the transgender character Anna Madrigal; the production is based on a novel by Armistead Maupin.

1993   Minnesota becomes the first U.S. state to offer transgender people legal protection against discrimination.

1993   At the Michigan Womyn's Music Festival, transgender people protest their exclusion and create "Camp Trans" outside the festival grounds to protest the festival's policy of allowing only those assigned female gender at birth to attend.

1994   Founding of Transsexual Menace, a direct action group focused on inclusion, by Denise Anne Norris, Riki Anne Wilchins, and others.

1994   The Australian film *Priscilla Queen of the Desert* includes a transsexual woman, played by Terence Stamp, as one of its three main characters.

1995   Creation of GenderPAC, an American political advocacy group for transgender people.

1995   The transgender woman Tyra Hunter is refused emergency medical care in Washington, DC, due to her gender identity. Hunter dies as a result; her mother sues and in 1998 the hospital in question is found guilty of malpractice and negligence, and Hunter's mother is awarded $2.8 million as compensation for her death.

1996   The University of Iowa adds gender identity to its list of protected categories, thus outlawing discrimination on the basis of gender identity within the university.

1997	Alain Berliner's film *Ma vie en rose*, about a child who was assigned male gender at birth but insists that she is a girl, wins the Golden Globe for Best Foreign Film.
December 1997	An article by John Colapinto in *Rolling Stone* tells the story of David Reimer, one of John Money's most famous patients, revealing that many claims Money made about Reimer and his treatment were not true.
1998	Murder of Rita Hester, a transgender woman; the Transgender Day of Remembrance (TDOR) was begun by Gwendolyn Ann Smith to honor her and to commemorate all transgender people.
1998	Pedro Almodóvar's film *All about My Mother* includes a transgender character that plays a key role in the film's plot.
1998	The national organization Parents and Friends of Lesbians and Gays (PFLAG) votes to include gender identity in their mission.
1999	Creation of the National Transgender Advocacy Coalition in the United States.
1999	Barry Winchell, a soldier in the U.S. Army, is murdered by a fellow soldier due to his relationship with the male-to-female transgender person Calpernia Addams.
1999	The first Transgender Day of Remembrance is held in San Francisco; by 2002, about 70 communities were observing this day, which commemorates transgender people killed due to anti-trans violence.
1999	Death of Robert Eads, a transgender man, of ovarian cancer. Eads experienced difficulty in finding medical care for his condition due to his transgender status.
2000	Cisgender actress Hilary Swank wins the Academy Award for Best Actress for her portrayal of Brandon Teena, a transgender man who was murdered in Nebraska, in the feature film *Boys Don't Cry*. Chloe Sevigny is also nominated, for Best Supporting Actress, for her portrayal of Teena's girlfriend Lana Tisdel.
2000	Dr. Jorge Daaboul delivers a lecture at the annual conference of the American Association for the History of Medicine arguing that, in the view of contemporary medical practice, an intersex individual could only achieve happiness and psychological adjustment by choosing either a male or female identity, rather than claiming an intersex identity.
2001	Rhode Island becomes the second U.S. state, after Minnesota, to offer legal protection from discrimination to transgender people.

2001	*The Education of Max Bickford*, the first American television program to include a transgender character, begins airing on CBS.
2002	Founding of the Transgender Law Center (TLC) in Oakland, California.
2002	Founding of the Sylvia Rivera Law Project in New York City, to provide legal services to transgender people in three main areas: survival and self-determination (e.g., name changes, healthcare advocacy), immigrant rights, and prisoner justice.
2002	Founding of the Transgender Law Center in San Francisco; a civil right organization, the Transgender Law Center advocates for the rights of transgender people.
2003	Founding of the Transgender American Veterans Association.
2003	In Mexico, Amaranta Gómez runs for Congress, making her the first transgender woman in Mexico to do so.
2003	Jennifer Finney Boylan, a transgender woman, publishes *She's Not There: A Life in Two Genders*, which becomes a bestseller.
2003	Founding of the National Center for Transgender Equality (NCTE) in Washington, DC. The NCTE is an advocacy organization working to change laws and policies at the local, state, and federal level.
2003	Mexico adds sexual orientation as a category protected from discrimination in categories including employment, education, property rights, and medical services.
2003	The International Olympic Committee requires transgender athletes to have reassignment surgery and two years of hormone treatment before being allowed to compete in the category indicated by their gender identity.
2004	In Great Britain, the Gender Recognition Act gives transgender people the right to acquire a birth certificate reflecting their gender identity and to marry and enjoy other sex-based social privileges based on their gender identity.
2005	California passes the Insurance Gender Nondiscrimination Act, making it the first state to mandate that transgender health be covered by health insurance companies.
2005	Cisgender actress Felicity Huffman is nominated for an Academy Award for her portrayal of the transgender character Bree in *Transamerica*.
2006	Kim Coco Iwamoto is elected to the Hawaii Board of Education, making her at the time the highest-ranking transgender

person elected to a government position in the United States; she was also the first openly transgender elected to a state-wide office.

2006	In Spain, the law is changed so that transgender people can change their gender in public documents without having to undergo surgery.
2006	On the HBO television program *The L Word*, first appearance of the transgender character Moira/Max (Daniela Sea), who is in the process of transitioning from female to male.
2007	Candis Cayne becomes the first transgender actress to play a recurring transgender character on American primetime television, on the drama *Dirty Sexy Money*.
2007	Transgender woman Theresa Sparks is elected president of the San Francisco Police Commission.
2007	Boston Children's Hospital in Massachusetts opens the Gender Management Service clinic, the first clinic in the nation founded to treat transgender children.
2008	The United Methodist Church in the United States votes down a motion that would have prohibited transgender people from serving as clergymen in the church.
2008	Trans woman Isis King is featured on the reality television program *America's Top Model*, making her the first transgender person to compete in the show, and as a result raising awareness of transgender people in the United States.
2008	An Islamic boarding school for transgender students, Pesantren Waria, is opened on the Indonesian island of Java.
2008	Diane Schroer wins a lawsuit filed against the Library of Congress; Schroer had been offered a job as a terrorism analyst, which was revoked when it became known that she was a transgender person, a decision that a judge determined was a violation of Title VII of the Civil Rights Act.
July 17, 2008	Trans woman Angie Zapata is murdered in Greeley, Colorado. The following year her killer, Allen Andrade, becomes the first person in the United States to be convicted of a hate crime involving a transgender person.
November 2008	Trans woman Stu Rasmussen is elected mayor of Silverton, Oregon, becoming the first transgender person to serve as mayor of an American city.
2009	France begins to allow transgender people to change their legal gender.
2009	South Burlington High School senior Kyle Giard-Chase advocates for the creation of gender-neutral bathrooms in Vermont Public Schools.

2009	Indonesia creates a Koran school in Yogyakarta for transgender students.
2009	Diego Michael Sanchez joins the staff of Representative Barney Frank of Massachusetts, making Sanchez the first openly transgender person to work on Capitol Hill.
2009–2013	About 150 universities in the United States install gender-neutral bathrooms on campus.
2010	The U.S. federal government includes gender identity among protected categories for federal employees, meaning that transgender people will have protection from discrimination on the same basis as is offered for discrimination on the basis of gender, race, and so on.
2010	Amanda Simpson is appointed to the post of senior technical advisor in the Bureau of Industry and Security within the Commerce Department, making her the first transgender person to be appointed by the president to a position in the federal government.
2010	Phyllis R. Frye becomes the first openly transgender judge in the United States after being appointed an associate judge for the city of Houston Municipal Courts.
2011	The Veterans Health Administration (VHA) in the United States declares that transgender veterans are entitled to be treated without discrimination at all VHA healthcare facilities.
2011	Cisgender actresses Glenn Close and Janet McTeer are nominated for Academy Awards (Best Actress and Best Supporting Actress, respectively) for their roles as transgender women in the British-Irish film *Albert Nobbs*, based on a novella by George Moore.
2011	CeCe McDonald, an African American trans woman, is arrested after killing a man who attacked her. In 2012, McDonald accepted a plea bargain for a 41-month sentence and was housed in several male prisons; her case draws national attention to the risks and injustices faced by transgender people.
2011	The Girl Scouts of America announces that anyone who identifies and presents as a girl and is in kindergarten through 12th grade may become a member.
2011	A census in India finds that almost half a million people self-identify as hijra.
January 2011	*Becoming Chaz*, a documentary directed by Fenton Bailey and Randy Barbato about the transition of Chaz Bono (born

Chastity Bono, to the American singing duo Sonny and Cher), premieres at the Sundance Film Festival.

2012   In Australia, the High Court rules that two transgender men did not need to undergo sterilization in order to obtain a gender recognition certificate; both had already had mastectomies and hormone treatment.

2012   Jenna Talackova becomes the first transgender person to compete in the Miss Universe Canada beauty pageant.

2012   First appearance of the transgender character "Unique Adams," played by Alex Newell, on the American television program *Glee*. Unique is reveled to be a transgender woman who is harassed by some of the other students.

2012   Transgender woman Laura Jane Grace, founder of the band Against Me, becomes the first major rock star to publicly identify as transgender.

2012   A transgender woman, Beth Scott, wins an appeal against her health insurer, Aetna, which had refused to pay for her to have a mammogram. Aetna later declared that they would not impose barriers to sex-specific care based on an individual's sex as recorded at birth or as recorded in their insurance records.

June 2012   Kylar Broadus becomes the first transgender person to testify before the U.S. Congress.

2012   The Equal Employment Opportunity Commission in the United States rules that discrimination based on gender identity constitutes gender-based discrimination and is therefore a violation of Title VII.

2013   California becomes the first state in the United States to require that students in public schools must be allowed to use facilities and participate in sex-segregated activities, including sports, based on gender identity, even if that identity conflicts with his or her gender as assigned at birth.

2013   Nikki Sinclaire becomes the first openly gay person serving in the Parliament of the United Kingdom.

2013   A poll conducted by the Pew Research Center found that, among the 43 transgender adults included in the sample, most said that they felt a discrepancy between their gender assigned at birth and their gender identity before puberty.

2013   In Australia, the Family Court of Australia rules that a 12-year-old who identifies as a girl but was assigned male gender at birth has the right to receive puberty blockers to prevent the development of secondary male sexual characteristics.

2013	The fifth edition of the *Diagnostic and Statistical Manual* of the American Psychological Association, known as *DSM-5*, removes the term *gender identity disorder*, which is replaced with *gender dysphoria*.
2013	A poll conducted by the Pew Research Center found that most LGBT people surveyed believed there is no (21%) or little (59%) acceptance of transgender people in American society.
2014	Essay Anne Vanderbilt commits suicide after a story revealing her transgender status is published on the website Grantland. The website received strong criticism for the story, which was originally meant to focus on a golf club developed about Vanderbilt, but instead focused on her transgender identity.
2014	The Southern Baptist Convention in the United States approves a resolution requiring transgender people to repent before they can become members.
2014	A report from the European Union indicates that, based on survey data, 54 percent of transgender people felt they had been harassed or discriminated against in the previous year because they were perceived as transgender, with reports of harassment highest among those who were young, from lower income categories, or not in the workforce. In addition, 22 percent reported that they felt discriminated against when seeking health care in the previous year.
2014	The Indian Supreme Court establishes transgender as a legal identity category and required official documents to include a third gender option alongside male and female.
May 2014	Medicare, a publicly funded health insurance program for low income people in the United States, begins covering sex assignment surgery.
August 2014	Austin, Texas, approves a law requiring that single-occupancy bathrooms be identified as gender neutral and carry signs to that effect.
November 2014	A survey by the mental health charity Pace found that almost half (48%) of transgender people under age 26 in England have attempted suicide, and 30 percent have attempted suicide within the past year.
2015	"Bathroom surveillance" bills are introduced in the state legislatures of Florida, Kentucky, Missouri, and Texas, restricting people to using public bathrooms associated with their sex, ignoring gender identity, and defining an individual's sex as that assigned at birth, associated with their

	chromosomal makeup, or as noted on official identification documents.
2015	In India, Manobi Bandopadhyay becomes the first transgender college principal in the country, taking over the leadership of Krishnagar Women's College in West Bengal.
2015	State legislatures in South Dakota and Minnesota introduce bills that would prohibit transgender student from participating on school sports teams based on their gender identity, if it is different from their sex as assigned at birth.
2015	In India, trans woman Rudrani Chettri Chauhan creates a modeling agency, Bold, for transgender people.
2015	State legislatures in Connecticut and South Carolina introduce legislation that would allow insurance companies to deny coverage of medically necessary health care to transgender people.
2015	Nineteen countries in Europe, including France, Belgium, Norway, and Italy, require that transgender people undergo medical intervention before being allowed to change their gender legally.
2015	The Union for Reform Judaism in the United States approves a resolution affirming their commitment to including and accepting transgender and gender nonconforming people.
2015	Riley Carter Millington, a transgender actor, is cast in the role of "Kyle" on the long-running British television program *EastEnders*.
January 20, 2015	President Barack Obama becomes the first American president to mention transgender people in a State of the Union Address, condemning the persecution of transgender people in the same sentence as condemning the persecution of women, religious minorities, and lesbian, gay, and bisexual people.
January 23, 2015	Sean S. Baker's film *Tangerine*, starring Kitana Kiki Rodriguez and Mya Taylor as transgender sex workers, opens to broad acclaim at the Sundance Film Festival.
February 2015	Laverne Cox, a trans woman who plays the character Sophia on the Netflix series *Orange Is the New Black*, becomes the first transgender person to be nominated for an Emmy Award.
March 2015	Sweden adds a gender-neutral pronoun to the official dictionary of the Swedish language.
March 2015	Madhu Kinnar, a transgender woman, is elected mayor of Raigarh, making her the only transgender mayor in India.

April 2015	The White House opens its first gender-neutral bathroom.
May 2015	Smith College, a women's college in Massachusetts, announces that it will admit transgender women as well as individuals who have been female from birth.
June 2015	Trans woman Caitlyn Jenner appears on the cover of *Vogue* magazine. Formerly Bruce Jenner, who gained fame as an Olympic decathlon champion, Jenner also discussed her transition in an article in the same issue.
June 2015	Barnard College, a women's college in New York City, votes to admit transgender women as well as women who have been female from birth.
July 2015	The Pentagon announces that it will lift a ban on transgender people serving in the military by 2016.
July 2015	Asher O'Callaghan, a transgender man, is ordained by the Evangelical Lutheran Church of America, the first openly transgender person to become a minster within this church.
July 2015	The U.S. Department of Justice rules in favor of Virginia high school student Galvin Grimm, stating that he can use the school bathroom that corresponds to his gender identity.
September 2015	The city of Philadelphia requires single-occupancy bathrooms to be gender neutral and to carry signage to that effect.
October 2015	A poll conducted by the Pew Research Institute with a nationally representative sample of teenagers aged 13 through 17 finds that 3 percent identify as transgender.
November 2015	The Tavistock and Portman NHS trust gender identity development service, the only NHS specialist service provider of gender identity support for people younger than 18, reports that the number of children seeking referrals has doubled over the previous six months.
November 2015	In France, a bill is introduced into the Senate that would allow transgender people to change their gender on legal documents without having to undergo sterilization; as of 2016, the bill was still going through the legislative process.
December 2015	Transgender couple Fernando Machado and Diane Rodriguez announce that they are expecting a baby, whose birth would make them the first transgender couple in Ecuador to become parents.
December 2015	Washington State clarifies that state law allows people to use public bathrooms based on their gender identity.
2016	The U.S. Department of Justice issues guidelines forbidding correction institutions from placing prisoners into units solely on the basis of their gender assignment at birth.

January 2016	The International Olympic Committee rules that transgender athletes can compete in international events, including the Olympics, without undergoing surgery. Those transitioning from female to male have no requirements to meet before competition, while those transitioning from male to female will have to demonstrate that the testosterone level has been below a specified level for at least one year before being allowed to compete.
January 2016	An endowed academic chair for transgender studies is created at the University of Victoria in British Columbia, Canada, funded by Jennifer Pritzker; Aaron Devor is the first to hold the chair.
February 2016	The Australian Bureau of Statistics includes a third category, "other," for gender, in addition to "male" and "female," for the 2016 census.
February 2016	The city of Charlotte, North Carolina, passes legislation allowing transgender people to use public bathrooms based on their gender identity.
March 2016	The state legislature of North Carolina passes HB2, the Public Facilities Privacy and Security Act, which restricts people to using only those public bathrooms that correspond with their gender as assigned at birth.
March 2016	Cooper Union, a college in New York City, begins removing gender designations from all its bathrooms.
March 2016	Dennis Daugaard, the governor of South Dakota, vetoes a bill that would have required students in public schools to use the bathrooms corresponding to their sex as assigned at birth.
April 2016	The BBC airs *Transgender: Back to Jamaica*, a half-hour film about two Jamaica-born transgender individuals who travel from Great Britain to Jamaica to reveal their new identities to their families.
May 2016	A poll in Australia conducted by ABC Vote Compass reveals that 46 percent of respondents do not believe transgender awareness should be taught in primary schools, while 37 percent believe it should be taught.
May 2016	Denmark's parliament decides to declassify being transgender as a mental illness, with the change to become active in 2017.
May 2016	Canada introduces legislation offering protection from discrimination and violence to transgender people.
May 2016	In the Philippines, Geraldine Roman becomes the first transgender person to be elected to the national congress.

May 2016	U.S. president Barack Obama orders all public schools in the United States to allow students to use the bathrooms that match their gender identities.
June 2016	An Oregon judge grants Jamie Shupe's request to be classified as gender nonbinary rather than male or female; this is the first time such a request has been upheld in the United States.
June 2016	Secretary of Defense Ash Carter announces that the United States will end the prohibition against transgender people serving in the military.
July 2016	A study published in the British medical journal *The Lancet* argues that being transgender should not be classified as a mental disorder, and that the distress experienced by some transgender people is due primarily to discrimination, violence, and social rejection, rather than being an inherent quality of being transgender.
July 2016	Ireland passes a bill allowing transgender people to change their legal status without having to undergo medical procedures or be diagnosed with a mental disorder.
July 2016	Sarah McBride speaks at the Democratic National Convention, becoming the first openly transgender person to address a major American political convention.
July 2016	A study of the 14 gender identity clinics operating in the United Kingdom found rapid increases in the number of patients treated in recent years. For instance, referrals at a clinic in Charing Cross, London, almost quadrupled (from 498 to 1,892) from 2006–2007 to 2015–2016, and a clinic in Nottingham reported a 28-fold increase in referrals, from 30 to 850, from 2008 to 2015.
August 2016	Legislation is introduced in Victoria, Australia, that would make it easier for people who change their gender to get a new birth certificate and no longer requires married people who change their gender to obtain a divorce.
August 2016	The United States experiences a national shortage of injectable estrogen in the two high-dosage formulations most commonly used by trans women.
August 2016	The murder of a transgender woman and LGBT activist, Hande Kader, in Istanbul, results in widespread protests.
September 2016	Cisgender male actor Jeffrey Tambour, in his speech after receiving an Emmy Award for his portrayal of a transgender woman in the Amazon series *Transparent*, called for more transgender actors to be considered for transgender roles.

October 2016	A survey of nursing staff in the United Kingdom finds that most (76%) have encountered a transgender person at work, 56 percent have directly cared for a transgender person, and of those who have provided direct care to a transgender person, 87 percent feel their training did not adequately prepare them to meet the needs of the patient(s).
October 2016	A number of investment groups, including Morgan Stanley and the New York State pension fund, publish a letter criticizing North Carolina's House Bill 2, which requires that transgender people only use the public bathrooms designated for their gender as assigned at birth rather than their current gender identity.
February 2017	Mack Beggs, a 17-year-old transgender boy, becomes a Texas state girls' wrestling champion. Beggs, who has stated that he would prefer to compete against boys, was about a year and a half into his transition at the time of the state championship.
June 13, 2017	Transgender politician Danica Roem is elected to the Virginia House of Delegates, making her the first openly transgender person to serve in any state legislature.
July 26, 2017	U.S. president Donald Trump issues a series of Tweets announcing that transgender people will no longer be allowed to serve in the U.S. military; he follows this up with a formal memorandum asking Secretary of Defense James Mattis to develop a plan to implement the ban by February 21, 2018.
January 22, 2018	The Oscar nominations for Best Documentary include *Strong Island*, directed by Yance Ford, making Ford the first transgender person to direct a film nominated for an Oscar.
February 2018	The Canadian Olympic Committee opens Pride House, a safe space for LGBTQ athletes and their supporters, at the 2018 Winter Olympics in South Korea.
February 14, 2018	A transgender woman in New York City is able to breastfeed her partner's child, making her the first documented case of successful induced lactation in a transgender woman. Physicians treated the woman using a system to promote lactation that is also used to induce lactation in women who have no given birth (e.g., who want to breastfeed an adopted child).
February 18, 2018	Transgender actor Daniela Vega is named as one of the presenters for the 2018 Oscars, making her the first openly transgender person to play that role in the ceremony.

Sources for Further Information

Books

American Psychiatric Association. *Diagnostic and Statistical Manual of Mental Disorders*. 5th ed. Arlington, VA: American Psychiatric Association, 2013. http://dsm.psychiatryonline.org/doi/book/10.1176/appi.books.97808904 25596 (accessed February 14, 2017).

Amnesty International. *The State Decides Who I Am: Lack of Legal Gender Recognition for Transgender People in Europe*. London: Amnesty International, 2014.

Australian Human Rights Commission. *Resilient Individuals: Sexual Orientation, Gender Identity & Intersex Rights: National Consultation Report 2015*. Sydney: Australian Human Rights Commission, 2015. https://www.human rights.gov.au/sites/default/files/document/publication/SOGII%20Rights%20 Report%202015_Web_Version.pdf (accessed September 1, 2016).

Beemyn, Genny, and Susan Rankin. *The Lives of Transgender People*. New York: Columbia University Press, 2011.

Bloom, Amy. *Normal: Transsexual CEOS, Crossdressing Cops, and Hermaphrodites with Attitude*. New York: Vintage, 2003.

Bockting, Walter, and Eric Avery, eds. *Transgender Health and HIV Prevention: Needs Assessment Studies from Transgender Communities across the United States*. New York: Haworth Medical Press, 2005.

Bourns, Jennifer. *Guidelines and Protocols for Hormone Therapy and Primary Health Care for Trans Clients*. Toronto: Rainbow Health Ontario, 2015. http://www.rainbowhealthontario.ca/wp-content/uploads/woocommerce_ uploads/2015/04/SHC-Protocols-for-Hormone-Therapy-Final1.pdf (accessed August 31, 2016).

Brill, Stephanie A., and Rachel Pepper. *The Transgender Child*. San Francisco, CA: Cleis Press, 2008.

Colapinto, John. *As Nature Made Him: The Boy Who Was Raised as a Girl.* New York: HarperCollins, 2000.

Deutsch, Madeline B., ed. *Guidelines for the Primary and Gender-Affirming Care of Transgender and Gender Nonbinary People.* 2nd ed. San Francisco, CA: Center of Excellence for Transgender Health, 2016. http://transhealth.ucsf .edu/pdf/Transgender-PGACG-6-17-16.pdf (accessed August 31, 2016).

Dohrenwent, Anne. *Coming Around: Parenting Lesbian, Gay, Bisexual, and Transgender Kids.* Far Hills, NJ: New Horizon Press, 2012.

Erickson-Schroth, Laura, ed. *Trans Bodies, Trans Selves: A Resource for the Transgender Community.* New York: Oxford University Press, 2014.

European Agency for Fundamental Human Rights. *Protection against Discrimination on Grounds of Sexual Orientation, Gender Identity and Sex Characteristics in the EU: Comparative Legal Analysis: Update 2015.* Luxembourg: Publications Office of the European Union, 2015. http://fra.europa.eu/ sites/default/files/fra_uploads/protection_against_discrimination_legal_ update_2015.pdf (accessed September 1, 2016).

European Union Agency for Fundamental Rights. *European Union Lesbian, Gay, Bisexual and Transgender Survey: Main Results.* Vienna: European Union Agency for Fundamental Rights, 2014. http://fra.europa.eu/sites/default/ files/fra-eu-lgbt-survey-main-results_tk3113640enc_1.pdf (accessed February 8, 2017).

Fausto-Sterling, Anne. *Sex/Gender: Biology in a Social World.* New York: Routledge, 2012.

Girschick, Lori B. *Transgender Voices: Beyond Women and Men.* Hanover: University Press of New England, 2009.

Grant, Jaime M., Lisa A. Mottet, and Justin Tanis. "Injustice at Every Turn: A Report of the National Transgender Discrimination Survey." Washington, DC: National Center for Transgender Equality and National Gay and Lesbian Task Force, 2011. http://www.thetaskforce.org/static_html/downloads/ reports/reports/ntds_full.pdf (accessed September 1, 2016).

Hanneman, Tari. HEI 2014: *Promoting Equitable and Inclusive Care for Lesbian, Gay, Bisexual and Transgender Patients and Their Families.* Washington, DC: Human Rights Campaign Foundation, 2014.

Herman, Jody L., ed. *Best Practices for Asking Questions to Identify Transgender and Other Gender Minority Respondents on Population-Based Surveys.* Los Angeles, CA: The Williams Institute, 2014. http://williamsinstitute.law.ucla .edu/wp-content/uploads/geniuss-report-sep-2014.pdf (accessed September 1, 2016).

Huegel, Kelly. *GLBTQ: The Survival Guide for Gay, Lesbian, Bisexual, Transgender, and Questioning Teens.* Rev. 2nd ed. Minneapolis, MN: Free Spirit Publications, 2011.

Human Rights Campaign. *Growing Up LGBT in America.* Washington, DC: Human Rights Campaign, 2012. http://www.hrc.org/youth-report/about-the-survey (accessed December 24, 2017).

Human Rights Watch. *A Changing Paradigm: US Medical Provider Discomfort with Intersex Care Practices.* New York: Human Rights Watch, 2017.

Humphreys, Laud. *Tearoom Trade: Impersonal Sex in Public Places.* Chicago: Aldine, 1970.

Institute of Medicine. *The Health of Lesbian, Gay, Bisexual, and Transgender People: Building a Foundation for Better Understanding.* Washington, DC: National Academies Press, 2011. http://www.ncbi.nlm.nih.gov/books/NBK64806/pdf/Bookshelf_NBK64806.pdf (accessed August 16, 2016).

James, Sandy E., Jody L. Herman, Susan Rankin, Mara Keisling, Lisa Mottet, and Ma'ayan Anafi. *The Report of the 2015 Transgender Survey.* Washington, DC: National Center for Transgender Equality, 2016. http://www.transequality.org/sites/default/files/docs/usts/USTS%20Full%20Report%20-%20FINAL%201.6.17.pdf (accessed February 7, 2017).

Jennings, Jazz. *Being Jazz: My Life as a (Transgender) Teen.* New York: Crown, 2016.

Kosciw, Joseph G., Emily A. Greytak, Noreen M. Giga, Christian Villenas, and David J. Danischewski. *The 2015 National School Climate Survey: The Experiences of Lesbian, Gay, Bisexual, Transgender, and Queer Youth in Our Nation's Schools.* New York: GLSEN, 2016. https://www.glsen.org/sites/default/files/2015%20National%20GLSEN%202015%20National%20School%20Climate%20Survey%20%28NSCS%29%20-%20Full%20Report.pdf (accessed February 13, 2017).

Kugle, Scott Alan. *Living Out Islam: Voices of Gay, Lesbian, and Transgender Muslims.* New York: New York University Press, 2013.

Kuklin, Susan. *Beyond Magenta: Transgender Teens Speak Out.* Somerville, MA: Candlewick Press, 2014.

Miyashita, Ayako, Amira Hasenbush, and Brad Sears. *The Legal Needs of Transgender Women Living with HIV: Evaluating Access to Justice in Los Angeles.* Los Angeles, CA: The Williams Institute, 2015.

Nodin, Nuno, Elizabeth Peel, Allan Tyler, and Ian Ribert. *The RaRE Research Report: LGB&T Mental Health—Risk and Resilience Explained.* London: PACE, 2015. https://uktrans.info/attachments/article/400/RARE_Research_Report_PACE_2015.pdf (accessed February 14, 2017).

Pan American Health Organization, John Snow, Inc., World Professional Association for Transgender Health et al. *Blueprint for the Provision of Comprehensive Care for Trans Persons and Their Communities in the Caribbean and Other Anglophone Countries.* Arlington, VA: John Snow, Inc., 2014. http://www.paho.org/hq/index.php?option=com_docman&task=doc_view&gid=28440&lang=en&Itemid=270 (accessed September 1, 2016).

Pepper, Rachel, ed. *Transitions of the Heart: Stories of Love, Struggle and Acceptance by Mothers of Transgender and Gender Variant Children.* Berkeley, CA: Cleis Press, 2012.

Radix, Anita, and Gal Mayer. "Lesbian, Gay, Bisexual, and Transgender Health: A Neglected Issue." In *Public Health in the 21st Century.* Vol. 1: Global

Issues in Public Health. Edited by Madelon L. Finkel, pp. 235–249. Santa Barbara, CA: Praeger, 2011.

Rupp, Leila J., and Susan K. Freeman, eds. *Understanding and Teaching U.S. Lesbian, Gay, Bisexual, and Transgender History.* Harvey Goldberg series for understanding and teaching history. Madison: University of Wisconsin Press, 2014.

Schultz, Jackson Wright. *Trans/Portraits: Voices from Transgender Communities.* Dartmouth, NH: Dartmouth College Press, 2015.

Skidmore, Emily. *True Sex: The Lives of Trans Men at the Turn of the Twentieth Century.* New York: New York University Press, 2017.

Stryker, Susan. *Transgender History: The Roots of Today's Revolution.* Berkeley, CA: Seal Press, 2008.

Substance Abuse and Mental Health Services Administration. *Top Health Issues of LGBT Populations: Information & Resource Kit.* HHS Public No. (SMA) 12–4684. Rockville, MD: SAMHSA, 2012.

United Nations Development Programme and the Williams Institute. *Surveying Nepal's Sexual and Gender Minorities: An Inclusive Approach.* Bangkok: UNDP, 2014.

Veale, J., E. Saewyc, H. Frohard-Dourlent, S. Dobson, B. Clark, and the Canadian Trans Youth Health Survey Research Group. *Being Safe, Being Me: Results of the Canadian Trans Youth Health Survey.* Vancouver, BC: Stigma and Resilience among Vulnerable Youth Centre, School of Nursing, University of British Columbia, 2015. http://saravyc.sites.olt.ubc.ca/files/2015/05/SARAVYC_Trans-Youth-Health-Report_EN_Final_Print.pdf (accessed February 13, 2017).

Whittington, Hillary, and Kristine Gasbarre. *Raising Ryland: Our Story of Parenting a Transgender Child with No Strings Attached.* New York: William Morrow, 2016.

ARTICLES

Aguayo-Romero, Natalie M. Alizaga, and Courtney Glickman. "The Dynamics of Intersectionality and Gender Affirmation on HIV Risk among Transgender IPV Survivors." *Psychology and AIDS Exchange Newsletter* (April 2016). http://www.apa.org/pi/aids/resources/exchange/2016/04/gender-affirmation.aspx (accessed February 7, 2017).

American Psychiatric Association. "What Is Gender Dysphoria?" (February 2016). https://www.psychiatry.org/patients-families/gender-dysphoria/what-is-gender-dysphoria (accessed February 14, 2017).

American Psychological Association. "Guidelines for Psychological Practice with Transgender and Gender Nonconforming People." *American Psychology* 70, no. 9 (December 2015): 832–864. http://www.apa.org/practice/guidelines/transgender.pdf (accessed August 31, 2016).

Bauer, Greta R., Ayden I. Scheim, Jake Pyne, Robb Travers, and Rebecca Hammond. "Intervenable Factors Associated with Suicide Risk in Transgender

Persons: A Respondent Driven Sampling Study in Ontario, Canada." *BMC Public Health* 15 (2015): 525. https://bmcpublichealth.biomedcentral.com/ articles/10.1186/s12889-015-1867-2 (accessed February 14, 2017).

Bazelon, Emily. "Cross-Court Winner." *Slate* (October 25, 2012). http://www .slate.com/articles/sports/sports_nut/2012/10/jewish_jocks_and_ren_e_rich ards_the_life_of_the_transsexual_tennis_legend.html (accessed February 19, 2018).

Benenson Strategy Group. "Report to Fusion.Net: January 2015 Poll of Millennials." https://fusiondotnet.files.wordpress.com/2015/02/fusion-poll-gender-spectrum.pdf (accessed February 13, 2018).

Blosnich, John R., George R. Brown, Jillian C. Shipherd, Michael Kauth, Rebecca I. Piegari, and Robert M. Bossarte. "Prevalence of Gender Identity Disorder and Suicide Risk among Transgender Veterans Utilizing Veterans Health Administration Care." *American Journal of Public Health* 103, no. 10 (October 2013): e27–e32. http://www.ncbi.nlm.nih.gov/pmc/articles/ PMC3780758/ (accessed August 16, 2016).

Brightwell, Laura. "Trans Health Care in Canada: A Provincial Lottery." Rabble. ca (June 29, 2016). http://rabble.ca/news/2016/06/trans-health-care-canada-provincial-lottery (accessed February 12, 2016).

Brown, Taylor N.T., and Jody L. Herman. "Voter ID Laws and Their Costs for Transgender Voters." The Williams Institute (March 2016). http://williamsinsti tute.law.ucla.edu/wp-content/uploads/Voter-ID-Laws-and-Their-Added-Costs-for-Transgender-Voters-March-2016.pdf (accessed September 1, 2016).

Cantor, James. "Do Trans-Kids Stay Trans When They Grow Up?" *Sexology Today* (January 2016). http://www.sexologytoday.org/2016/01/do-trans-kids-stay-trans-when-they-grow_99.html (accessed February 14, 2017).

Coleman, Todd, Greta Bauer, Kyle Scanlon, Robb Travers, Matthias Kaay, and Matt Francino. "Challenging the Binary: Gender Characteristics of Trans Ontarians." *Trans PULSE E-Bulletin* 2, no. 2 (December 15, 2011). http://www.rainbowhealthontario.ca/wp-content/uploads/woocommerce_ uploads/2014/08/trans%20health%20findings%20English.pdf (accessed August 31, 2016).

Crenshaw, Kimberle. "Mapping the Margins: Intersectionality, Identity Politics, and Violence against Women of Color." *Stanford Law Review* 43 (July 1991): 1241–1299. http://socialdifference.columbia.edu/files/socialdiff/projects/ Article__Mapping_the_Margins_by_Kimblere_Crenshaw.pdf (accessed February 7, 2017).

Cutler, Anne, and Donia R. Scott. "Speaker Sex and Perceived Apportionment of Talk." *Applied Linguistics* 11 (1990): 253–272.

Dickey, Lore M., Michael L. Hendricks, and Walter O. Bockting. "Innovations in Research with Transgender and Gender Nonconforming People and Their Communities." *Psychology of Sexual Orientation and Gender Identity* 3, no. 3 (2016): 187–194.

Dickey, Lore M, Sabra L. Katz-Wise, Stephanie L. Budge, and Michael V. Garza. "Disparities in the Transgender Community: Exploring Differences in Insurance Coverage." *Psychology of Sexual Orientation and Gender Identity* 3, no. 3 (2016): 275–282.

Drescher, Jack, Alan Schwartz, Flavio Casoy, Christopher A. McIntosh, Brian Hurley, Kenneth Ashley, Mary Barber et al. "The Growing Regulation of Conversion Therapy." *Journal of Medical Regulation* 102, no. 2 (2016): 7–12. https://www.ncbi.nlm.nih.gov/pmc/articles/PMC5040471/pdf/nihms815682 .pdf (accessed February 14, 2017).

Erich, Stephen, Josephine Tittsworth, Janice Dykes, and Charyl Cabuses. "Family Relationship and Their Correlations with Transsexual Well-Being." *Journal of GLBT Family Studies* 4, no. 4 (2008): 419–432.

Fausto-Sterling, Anne. "The Five Sexes: Why Male and Female Are Not Enough." *The Sciences* (March/April 1993): 20–25.

Flores, Andrew R., Jody L. Herman, Gary J. Gates, and Taylor N.T. Brown. "How Many Adults Identify as Transgender in the United States?" The Williams Institute (June 2016). http://williamsinstitute.law.ucla.edu/wp-content/ uploads/How-Many-Adults-Identify-as-Transgender-in-the-United-States .pdf (accessed September 1, 2016).

Gates, Gary J. "How Many People Are Lesbian, Gay, Bisexual, and Transgender?" The Williams Institute (2011). http://williamsinstitute.law.ucla.edu/ wp-content/uploads/Gates-How-Many-People-LGBT-Apr-2011.pdf (accessed September 1, 2016).

Gates, Gary J., and Jody L. Herman. "Transgender Military Service in the United States." Williams Institute (2014). http://williamsinstitute.law.ucla.edu/wp-content/uploads/Transgender-Military-Service-May-2014.pdf (accessed September 1, 2016).

Glicksman, Eve. "Transgender Today." *Monitor on Psychology* 44, no. 4 (April 13, 2013): 36. http://www.apa.org/monitor/2013/04/transgender.aspx (accessed October 24, 2017).

Haas, Anne P., Philip L. Rodgers, and Jody L. Herman. "Suicide Attempts among Transgender and Gender Nonconforming Adults: Findings of the National Transgender Discrimination Survey." (American Foundation for Suicide Prevention and the Williams Institute (January 2014). http://williamsinstitute .law.ucla.edu/wp-content/uploads/AFSP-Williams-Suicide-Report-Final.pdf (accessed September 1, 2016).

Harris, Benjamin Cerf. "Likely Transgender Individuals in U.S. Federal Administrative Records and the 2010 Census." CARRA Working Paper #015–03. Washington, DC: Center for Administrative Records Research and Applications, U.S. Census Bureau, 2015. "Likely Transgender Individuals in U.S. Federal Administrative Records and the 2010 Census." https://www .census.gov/srd/carra/15_03_Likely_Transgender_Individuals_in_ARs_ and_2010Census.pdf (accessed February 13, 2017).

Heggie, Vanessa. "Testing Sex and Gender in Sports: Reinventing, Reimagining, and Reconstructing Histories." *Endeavour* 34, no. 4 (December 2010): 157–163.

Herman, Jody L. "Costs and Benefits of Providing Transition-Related Health Care Coverage in Employee Health Benefits Plans: Findings from a Survey of Employers." The Williams Institute (September 2013). http://williams institute.law.ucla.edu/wp-content/uploads/Herman-Cost-Benefit-of-Trans-Health-Benefits-Sept-2013.pdf (accessed September 1, 2016).

Herman, Jody L. "Gendered Restrooms and Minority Stress: The Public Regulation of Gender and Its Impact on Transgender People's Lives." *Journal of Public Management & Social Policy* 19 (Spring 2013): 65–80. http://williams institute.law.ucla.edu/wp-content/uploads/Herman-Gendered-Restrooms-and-Minority-Stress-June-2013.pdf (accessed September 1, 2016).

Herzog, Katie. "The Detransitioners: They Were Transgender, Until They Weren't." *The Stranger* (June 28, 2017). https://www.thestranger.com/fea tures/2017/06/28/25252342/the-detransitioners-they-were-transgender-until-they-werent (accessed December 24, 2017).

Kirby, Andrew. "Freud on Homosexuality." *Psychotherapy Papers* [n.d.] https://psychotherapypapers.wordpress.com/2008/11/12/kirby1/ (accessed February 13, 2017).

Lambda Legal, Human Rights Campaign Foundation, Hogan Lovells, and the New York City Bar. Transgender-Affirming Hospital Policies: Creating Equal Access to Quality Health Care for Transgender Patients. (Rev. May 2016). http://www.lambdalegal.org/publications/fs_transgender-affirming-hospital-policies (accessed February 21, 2016).

MacNell, Lillian, Adam Driscoll, and Andrea N. Hunt. "What's in a Name: Exposing Gender Bias in Student Ratings of Teaching." *Innovative Higher Education* 40, no. 4 (August 2015): 291–303.

Marcellin, Roxanne Longman, Ayden Scheim, Greta Bauer, and Nik Redman. "Experiences of Transphobia among Trans Ontarians." *Trans PULSE E-Bulletin* 3, no. 2 (March 7, 2013). http://www.rainbowhealthontario.ca/wp-content/uploads/woocommerce_uploads/2014/08/Transphobia-E-Bulle tin-6-vFinal-English.pdf (accessed August 31, 2016).

Martin, James I., and William Meezan. "Applying Ethical Standards to Research and Evaluations Involving Lesbian, Gay, Bisexual, and Transgender Populations." *Journal of Gay & Lesbian Social Services* 15, no. 1–2 (2003/2004): 181–201.

Moss-Racusin, Corrine A., John F. Dovidio, Victoria L. Brescoll, Mark J. Graham, and Jo Handelsman. "Science Faculty's Subtle Gender Biases Favor Male Students." *Proceedings of the National Academy of Sciences* (September 17, 2012). http://www.pnas.org/content/early/2012/09/14/1211286109 (accessed February 12, 2018).

Poteat, Tonia, Ayden Scheim, Jessica Xavier, Sari Reisner, and Stefan Baral. "Global Epidemiology of HIV Infection and Related Syndemics Affecting Transgender People." *Journal of Acquired Immune Deficiency Syndromes* 72, Suppl. 3 (2016): S210–S219.

Potter, Jennifer, Sarah M. Peitzmeier, Ida Bernstein, Sari L. Reisner, Natalie M. Alizaga, Madina Agénor, and Dana J. Pardee. "Cervical Cancer Screening for Patients on the Female-to-Male Spectrum: A Narrative Review and Guide for Clinicians." *Journal of General Internal Medicine* 30, no. 12 (December 2015): 1857–1864. http://link.springer.com/article/10.1007/s11606-015-3462-8 (accessed August 31, 2016).

Rhodan, Maya. "Obamacare Rule Bans Discrimination against Transgender Patients." *Time* 187 (May 13, 2016). http://time.com/4329609/transgender-discrimination-obamacare-healthcare/ (accessed September 1, 2016).

Schaefer, Agnes Gereben, Radja Iyengar, Srikanth Kadiyala, Jennifer Kavanagh, Charles C. Engel, Kayla M. Williams, and Amii M. Kress. "Assessing the Implications of Allowing Transgender Personnel to Serve Openly." (RAND Corporation, 2016). https://www.rand.org/pubs/research_reports/RR1530 .html (accessed December 24, 2017).

Scheim, Ayden I., Gelnn-Milo Santos, Sonya Arreola, Keletso Makofane, Tri D. Do, Patrick Hebert, Matthew Thomann, and George Ayala. "Inequities in Access to HIV Prevention Services for Transgender Men: Results of a Global Survey of Men Who Have Sex with Men." *Journal of the International AIDS Society* 19, Suppl. 2 (2016): 20779. http://www.jiasociety.org/index.php/jias/ article/view/20779/pdf_1 (accessed September 1, 2016).

Schilt, Kristen, and Matthew Wiswall. "Before and After: Gender Transitions, Human Capital, and Workplace Experiences." *B.E. Journal of Economic Analysis and Policy* 8, no. 1 (2008): 39. https://www.ilga-europe.org/sites/ default/files/before_and_after_-_gender_transitions_human_capital_and_ workplace.pdf (accessed October 24, 2017).

Spade, Dean. "Documenting Gender." *Hasting Law Journal* 59 (2008): 731–842. http://williamsinstitute.law.ucla.edu/wp-content/uploads/Spade-Document ing-Gender-Apr-2008.pdf (accessed September 1, 2016).

Stolzer, Rebecca L., Jody L. Herman, and Amira Hasenbush. "Transgender Parenting: A Review of Existing Research." The Williams Institute (October 2014). http://williamsinstitute.law.ucla.edu/wp-content/uploads/transgender-parenting-oct-2014.pdf (accessed September 1, 2016).

Sullivan, Gerald, and Warren Losberg. "A Study of Sampling in Research in the Field of Lesbian and Gay Studies." *Journal of Gay & Lesbian Social Services* 15, no. 1–2 (2003): 147–162.

Taylor, Chris. "Transgender Surgery Can Cost More Than $100,000." Reuters 186 (October 29, 2015). http://time.com/money/4092680/transgender-surgery-costs/?xid=tcoshare (accessed September 1, 2016).

Taylor, Marisa. "First VA Clinic for Transgender Vets in US Opens in Ohio." *Aljazeera America* (November 12, 2015). http://america.aljazeera.com/arti cles/2015/11/12/ohio-va-opens-clinic-for-trans-veterans.html (accessed September 1, 2016).

Thomsen-Reuters. "Canadian Government Considering Gender-Neutral ID." *CBC News* (July 3, 2016). http://www.cbc.ca/news/canada/gender-neutral-id-1.3663111 (accessed February 8, 2017).

Transgender Europe. "Trans Murder Monitoring 2015" (2015). http://tgeu.org/tmm-idahot-update-2015/ (accessed September 1, 2016).

Transgender Europe. "Trans Rights Europe Map & Index 2016." (May 10, 2016). http://tgeu.org/trans-rights_europe_map_2016/ (accessed September 1, 2016).

Vanderbilt University School of Medicine, Program for LGBTI Health. "Key Transgender Health Concerns." (2012). https://www.vumc.org/lgbti/key-transgender-health-concerns (accessed February 22, 2017).

Wheeler, Darrell P. "Methodological Issues in Conducting Community-Based Health and Social Services Research among Urban Black and African American LGBT Populations." *Journal of Gay and Lesbian Social Services: Issues in Practice, Policy, and Research* 15, no. 1–2 (2003): 65–78.

Wiewel, Ellen Weiss, Lucia V. Torian, Pooja Merchant, Sarah L. Braunstein, and Colin W. Shepart. "HIV Diagnoses and Care among Transgender Persons and Comparison with Men Who Have Sex with Men: New York City, 2006–2011." *American Journal of Public Health* 106, no. 3 (March 2016): 497–502.

Winter, Sam, Milton Diamong, Jamison Green, Dan Karasic, Terry Reed, Stephen Whittle, and Kevan Wylie. "Transgender People: Health at the Margins of Society." *The Lancet* 388 (2016): 390–400. http://www.thelancet.com/pdfs/journals/lancet/PIIS0140-6736(16)00683-8.pdf (accessed February 12, 2017).

Workowski, Kimberly A., and Gail A. Bolan. "Sexually Transmitted Diseases Treatment Guidelines, 2015." *Morbidity and Mortality Weekly Report* 64, RR3 (June 5, 2015): 1–137. http://www.cdc.gov/mmwr/preview/mmwrhtml/rr6403a1.htm (accessed September 1, 2016).

World Health Organization. *Transgender People and HIV*. Policy Brief (July 2015). http://apps.who.int/iris/bitstream/10665/179517/1/WHO_HIV_2015.17_eng.pdf?ua=1&ua=1 (accessed February 15, 2017).

World Professional Association for Transgender Health. "WPATH Clarification on Medical Necessity of Treatment, Sex Reassignment, and Insurance Coverage in the U.S.A." (2008). http://www.tgender.net/taw/WPATHMedNecofSRS.pdf (accessed September 1, 2016).

WEBSITES

Asia-Pacific Transgender Network. http://www.weareaptn.org (accessed September 1, 2016).

Black Transmen, Inc. http://blacktransmen.org (accessed August 31, 2016).

Centers for Disease Control and Prevention. Lesbian, Gay, Bisexual, and Transgender Health. http://www.cdc.gov/lgbthealth/transgender.htm (accessed August 16, 2016).

Center of Excellence for Transgender Health, University of California, San Francisco. http://transhealth.ucsf.edu (accessed August 16, 2016).

Centers for Disease Control and Prevention. Lesbian, Gay, Bisexual, and Transgender Health. http://www.cdc.gov/lgbthealth/transgender.htm (accessed August 16, 2016).

European Union Agency for Fundamental Rights: LGBTI. http://fra.europa.eu/en/theme/lgbti (accessed September 1, 2016).

FTM International. http://www.ftmi.org (accessed August 31, 2016).

Gender Proud. http://genderproud.com/advocacy/ (accessed August 31, 2016).

Gender Spectrum. https://www.genderspectrum.org (accessed August 31, 2016).

GLAAD: Transgender Media Program. http://www.glaad.org/transgender (accessed August 31, 2016).

GLAD: Transgender Rights Project. http://www.glad.org/work/initiatives/c/trans gender-rights-project/ (accessed August 31, 2016).

GLMA: Health Professionals Advancing LGBT Equality. http://www.glma.org/index.cfm?fuseaction=Page.viewPage&pageId=532 (accessed August 16, 2016).

International Foundation for Gender Education. http://www.ifge.org (accessed August 31, 2016).

Massachusetts Transgender Political Coalition. http://www.masstpc.org (accessed August 31, 2016).

National Center for Transgender Equality. http://www.transequality.org (accessed August 16, 2016).

National LGBT Cancer Project. http://www.lgbtcancer.org (accessed August 31, 2016).

National LGBT Health Education Center, Fenway Institute. http://www.lgbtheal theducation.org (accessed August 16, 2016).

National LGBTQ Task Force. http://www.thetaskforce.org/transgender-activ ist-accuses-nypd-of-mistreatment-at-occupy-wall-street-protest/ (accessed August 31, 2016).

NHS Choices: Transgender Health. http://www.nhs.uk/Livewell/Transhealth/Pages/Transhealthhome.aspx (accessed September 1, 2016).

Rainbow Health Ontario/Santé arc-en-ciel Ontario: Resources. http://www.rain bowhealthontario.ca/resource-search/ (accessed August 31, 2016).

The Sylvia Rivera Law Project. http://srlp.org (accessed August 31, 2016).

Trans Latina Coalition. http://www.translatinacoalition.org (accessed August 31, 2016).

Trans People of Color Coalition. http://transpoc.org (accessed August 31, 2016).

Trans Student Educational Resources. http://www.transstudent.org (accessed August 31, 2016).

Trans Youth Equality Federation. http://www.transyouthequality.org (accessed August 31, 2016).

Transgender Europe. http://tgeu.org (accessed September 1, 2016).

Transgender Health [open-access journal]. http://www.liebertpub.com/overview/transgender-health/634/ (accessed August 16, 2016).

The Transgender, Gender Variant & Intersex Justice Project. http://www.tgijp.org (accessed August 31, 2016).

Transgender Health [open-access journal]. http://www.liebertpub.com/overview/transgender-health/634/ (accessed August 16, 2016).

Transgender Law and Policy Institute. http://www.transgenderlaw.org (accessed August 31, 2016).

Transgender Law Center. http://transgenderlawcenter.org (accessed August 31, 2016).

TransHealth. http://www.trans-health.com/ (accessed August 31, 2016).

TransLaw: Trans Legal Advocates of Washington. http://www.translawdc.org (accessed August 31, 2016).

TransYouth Family Allies. http://www.imatyfa.org (accessed August 31, 2016).

The Trevor Project. http://www.thetrevorproject.org (accessed August 31, 2016).

U.S. Department of Veterans Affairs, Lesbian, Gay, Bisexual and Transgender (LGBT) Veteran Care. http://www.patientcare.va.gov/LGBT/index.asp (accessed September 1, 2016).

United Nations Free & Equal. https://www.unfe.org (accessed September 1, 2016).

World Professional Association for Transgender Health. http://www.wpath.org (accessed September 1, 2016).

PAMPHLETS

Allison, Rebecca A. "Ten Things Transgender Persons Should Discuss with Their Healthcare Provider." (GLMA, May 2012). http://www.health.umd.edu/sites/default/files/10%20things%20to%20discuss%20with%20provider_trans.PDF (accessed August 16, 2016).

American Lung Association. "Smoking Out a Deadly Threat: Tobacco Use in the LGBT Community." (2010). http://www.lung.org/assets/documents/research/lgbt-report.pdf (accessed August 16, 2016).

American Psychological Association. "Answers to Your Questions about Transgender People, Gender Identity, and Gender Expression." Public and Member Communications 202.336.5700 (2011). http://www.apa.org/topics/lgbt/transgender.pdf (accessed September 1, 2016).

Bauer, Greta, and Ayden Scheim. "Transgender People in Ontario, Canada: Statistics from the Trans PULSE Project to Inform Human Rights Policy." (2015). http://www.rainbowhealthontario.ca/wp-content/uploads/woocommerce_uploads/2015/09/Trans-PULSE-Statistics-Relevant-for-Human-Rights-Policy-June-2015.pdf (accessed August 31, 2016).

Bhasin, Shalender, and Vin Tangpricha. "Patient Guide: Endocrine Treatment of Transsexual Persons." (Endocrine Society, 2016). http://www.hormone.org/patient-guides/2009/endocrine-treatment-of-transsexuals (accessed September 1, 2016).

Cooper, Charlotte, Margaret Robinson, and Loralee Gillis. "LGBTQ People and Exercise." (Rainbow Health Ontario/Santé arc-en-ciel Ontario, 2015).

http://www.rainbowhealthontario.ca/wp-content/uploads/woocommer
ce_uploads/2015/06/RHO_FactSheet_LGBTEXERCISE_E.pdf (accessed
August 31, 2016).

Laing, Marie. "Two-Spirit and LGBTQ Indigenous Health." (Rainbow Health
Ontario/Santé arc-en-ciel Ontario, 2016). http://www.rainbowhealthontario
.ca/wp-content/uploads/2016/07/2SLGBTQINDIGENOUSHEALTHFactH
eet.pdf (accessed August 31, 2016).

Orr, Asaf, and Joel Baum. "Schools in Transition: A Guide for Supporting Transgender Students in K-12 Schools." (2015). https://www.genderspectrum
.org/staging/wp-content/uploads/2015/08/Schools-in-Transition-2015.pdf
(accessed August 31, 2016).

Popowich, Dominic. "Intimate Partner Violence in LGBTQ Communities."
(Rainbow Health Ontario/Santé arc-en-ciel Ontario, 2016). http://www
.rainbowhealthontario.ca/wp-content/uploads/2016/07/RHO_FactSheet_
LGBTQIntimatePartnerViolence_E.pdf (accessed August 31, 2016).

Popowich, Dominic. "LGBTQ Cancer Factsheet" (Rainbow Health Ontario/Santé
arc-en-ciel Ontario, 2016). http://www.rainbowhealthontario.ca/wp-content/
uploads/woocommerce_uploads/2016/07/RHO_FactSheet_LGBTQCAN
CER_-07.31.16.pdf (accessed August 31, 2016).

Potter, M. "Tips for Providing Paps to Trans Men." (LGBT Family Health Team,
Sherbourne Health Center, n.d.). http://checkitoutguys.ca/sites/default/files/
Tips_Paps_TransMen_0.pdf (accessed August 31, 2016).

Pyne, Jake. "Supporting Gender Independent Children and Their Families."
(Rainbow Health Ontario/Santé arc-en-ciel Ontario, 2012). http://www.rain
bowhealthontario.ca/resources/page/10/?orderby=date (accessed August 31,
2016).

Robinson, Margaret. "LGBTQ People, Drug Use & Harm Reductions." (Rainbow
Health Ontario/Santé arc-en-ciel Ontario, 2014). http://www.rainbowhealth
ontario.ca/wp-content/uploads/woocommerce_uploads/2015/06/RHO_Fact
Sheet_LGBTDRUGUSEHARMREDUCTION_E.pdf (accessed August 31,
2016).

Terrence Higgins Trust. "Sexual Health, HIV and Wellbeing: A Guide for Trans
Men." (2012). http://www.rainbowhealthontario.ca/wp-content/uploads/woo
commerce_uploads/2014/08/Transmen%20THT.pdf (accessed August 31,
2016).

Terrence Higgins Trust. "Sexual Health, HIV and Wellbeing: A Guide for Trans
Women." (2012). http://www.rainbowhealthontario.ca/wp-content/uploads/
woocommerce_uploads/2014/08/Trans%20Women%20THT.pdf (accessed
August 31, 2016).

"Transition Options for Gender Independent Children and Adolescents: Information for Parent." (Rainbow Health Ontario, 2013). http://www.rainbow
healthontario.ca/wp-content/uploads/woocommerce_uploads/2014/08/Tran
sition%20Options%20Brochure.pdf (accessed August 31, 2016).

U.S. Department of Veterans Affairs. "Female Veterans: Transgender Female Health Care." http://www.patientcare.va.gov/LGBT/docs/va-pcs-lgbt-fact sheet-transgender-female.pdf# (accessed September 1, 2016).

U.S. Department of Veterans Affairs. "Male Veterans: Transgender Male Health Care." http://www.patientcare.va.gov/LGBT/docs/va-pcs-lgbt-factsheet-trans gender-male.pdf# (accessed September 1, 2016).

World Health Organization. "Gender." Fact Sheet No. 403 (August 2015). http://www.who.int/mediacentre/factsheets/fs403/en/ (accessed September 1, 2016).

World Health Organization. "Transgender People." http://www.who.int/hiv/top ics/transgender/en/ (accessed September 1, 2016).

INDEX

ABOUT THE AUTHOR

Sarah Boslaugh, PhD, MPH, has over 20 years of experience working as a statistical analyst in medicine and public health. Her previous books include *Statistics in a Nutshell, Healthcare Systems around the World: A Comparative Guide*, and *Drug Resistance* (ABC-CLIO); she also edited the *Encyclopedia of Epidemiology* and *The Encyclopedia of Pharmacology and Society* for Sage. In her spare time, she edits the film section of TheArtsStl, a popular culture publication based in Saint Louis, Missouri, and reviews books and films for PopMatters (www.popmatters.com) and TheArtsStl (www.theartsstl.com).